DALY BEAUTY

BARBARA DALY

Macdonald

Editor
Sam Hanson
Designer
Anthony Essam
Photographs
John Swannell
Hair
John Frieda
Styling
Annabel Hodin
Clothes
Emanuel
Jeff Banks
Juliet Dunn
Jewellery
Butler and Wilson

Illustrations
Alexander Vethers

For Macdonald Educational:
Editorial manager
Judy Maxwell
Senior editor
Neil Tennant
Editor
Bridget Daly
Production
John Moulder

Published in association with
Thames Television's programme
After Noon Plus edited by
Catherine Freeman.

First published 1980
Macdonald Educational Ltd
Holywell House
Worship Street
London EC2A 2EN

Made and printed by
Morrison and Gibb Limited
London and Edinburgh

ISBN 0 356 07179 0

CONTENTS

INTRODUCTION

Does the perfect face really exist? It is very doubtful and should it exist, it would be hard to describe, because the whole concept of beauty is directly related to the ever-changing face of fashion. But whatever that fashion, make-up is an art that is worth learning. That is what this book is all about – learning to see your face as a canvas, keeping that canvas in good condition and acquiring a fundamental knowledge of the most effective way of putting on the paint. Add to that knowledge a little bit of your own imagination and you can soon learn to make the most of your face.

If you look good, you feel good – that is a simple fact. And despite the fact that your husband, friend or lover tells you that you look terrific without all that stuff on your face, the majority of women gain a lot of confidence from their cosmetics. (Unless of course your friends are trying to tell you in a subtle way that you have overdone it a bit!) It is not always necessary to use masses of make-up, sometimes just a few products properly applied can be all you need.

I hope that you will enjoy this book and that it will teach you a little more about make-up and skin care than you knew before. The main thing is not to worry about the way that you look, just make the best of what you have and remember that no one is perfect!

Basic equipment

You do not need to spend a small fortune to kit yourself out. Firstly you will need your skin-care items which will usually consist of a cleanser, a toner and a moisturiser and, possibly, one or two additional items specifically for your skin type. A supply of tissues and cotton wool would be handy and a magnifying mirror is very useful – especially if you are short-sighted. You will also need a pair of eyebrow tweezers.

When it comes to choosing your make-up, bear in mind that, although types and colours vary according to individual choice, you will need several basic items: one foundation, one concealer (to cover spots or blemishes), a blusher, face powder, two or three eye colours, a mascara, one or two lipsticks and one lip gloss. This may look like a lot of cosmetics but you can build up your kit slowly and it is a good idea to include two or three make-up brushes, a baby sponge and a spare powder puff. All the cosmetics should fit comfortably into a make-up bag.

Storage

As you get better at dealing with your make-up, you will naturally experiment a little more with products and colours, some of which you will not want to carry around with you. However it is not a good idea to leave everything jumbled up in the bathroom or on your dressing table – this is how things get broken and spoiled. Take a tip from a professional and store your make-up neatly in a small tool box or a fishing-tackle case.

Once you have got the basic ingredients and learnt the techniques, you should be able to achieve the looks you want.

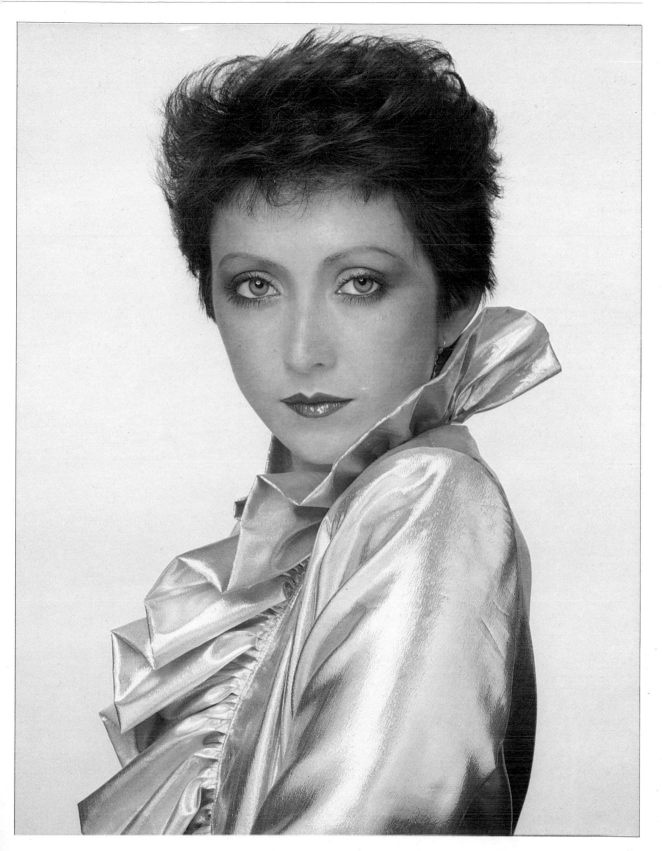

Light

Before you begin to re-think your skin care and beauty routines, get rid of all your pre-conceived notions. First of all think about where you are going to be when you put on your make-up. Yes, I do mean actually where you are going to be, because you cannot hope to make up properly if your face is literally in the dark!

Do not sit with the light on one side of you when putting on your make-up.

The right lighting is essential for a good make-up. If you are going out in the day time you should apply your make-up in daylight. If the

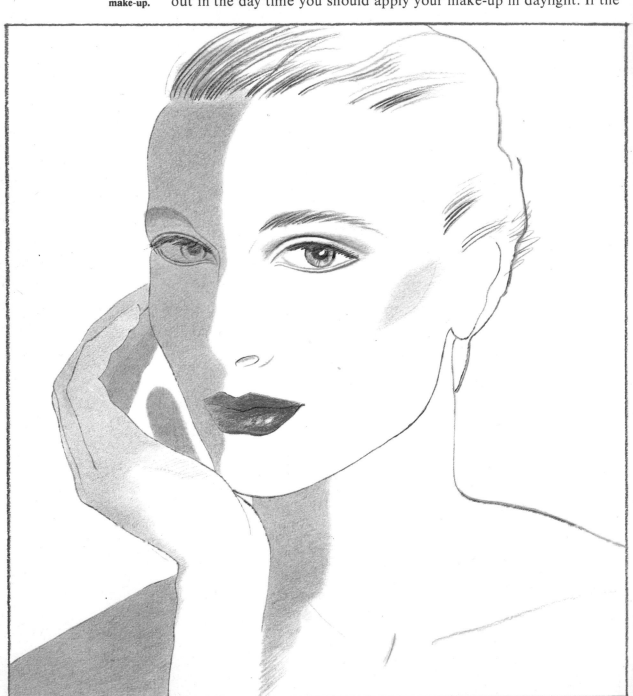

place where you make up is not directly in front of a window, take your make-up to the nearest source of daylight. Do not sit with the daylight falling on one side of you, make sure it falls directly on to your face. Whatever you do, even on dark winter mornings, do not fall into the trap of making up in a dim bathroom light. In the evening, it is best to put on your make-up in front of a direct light – you could simply take the shade off a lamp. So remember, always use the right light for the occasion, and you will avoid making major mistakes.

Do make sure that the light, whether natural or artificial, falls directly on to your face.

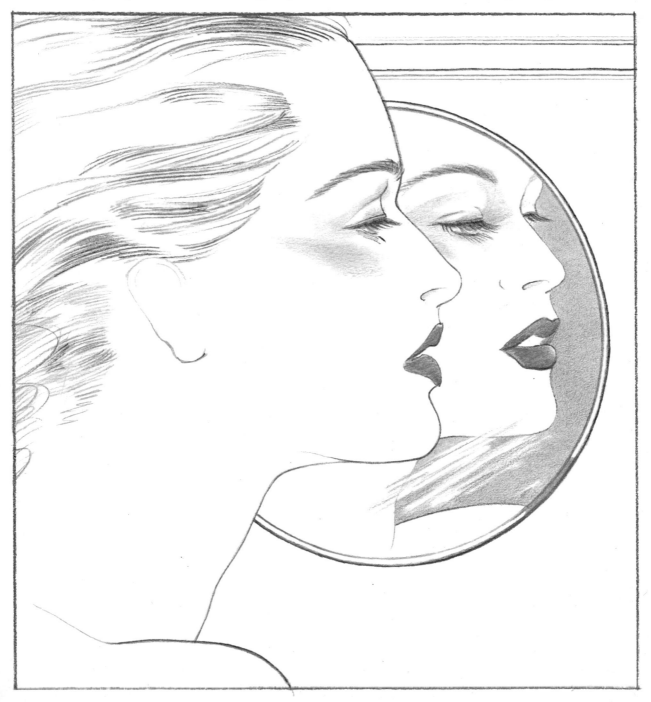

SKIN TYPES

Your skin is your own individual body suit, which has to last you a lifetime. You cannot buy a new one, so it is worth taking care of the one you have. Skin is a unique covering that is both germ-proof and waterproof and is constantly replacing itself. It does this by growing new cells from the bottom layers and sloughing off the old top layers.

The condition of your skin can reflect both your mental and physical states and you soon learn to recognize the signs when you are not feeling 100 per cent. Being under a lot of pressure or feeling low and depressed can adversely affect the way your skin looks. When you are feeling on top of the world your skin can look very good.

If you compare the skin on your hands and face with that on your body, you will find that your body skin is often much smoother, because it is usually protected by layers of clothing. Your face, throat and hands, however, are constantly exposed to the effects of the environment. So, let us start with the unavoidable truth or, to put it another way, the bad news. Air conditioning, central heating, dirty city air, exhaust fumes and cigarette smoke are all harmful to the skin. Even if you do not smoke, you may be surrounded by smokers, and your skin will suffer as much as theirs. Even fresh country air is not as fresh as it used to be!

The weather takes its toll on your skin as well. Everyone knows that skin needs protection in the sun, but this also applies to cold, wet, windy weather which can have just as bad an effect on your skin as too much sun. We all know the expression 'weather-beaten face' but nobody really wants flaking lined skin and chapped lips!

Another factor which inevitably affects skin is your age. With ageing, skin changes and loses both moisture and elasticity. Everyone has wrinkles – but no-one needs to have tram-lines. The key factor in this process is moisture, which keeps your skin supple. Using a moisturiser and cleansing skin properly helps to retain that moisture and keeps skin looking young. It is important to make a habit of looking after your skin as soon as possible because, although it may be very good when you are young, establishing a sensible routine will help to preserve that quality for longer.

It is also important to remember that your skin has the same composition all over. Some areas are more sensitive than others and some are tougher, but basically it is the same.

Body skin, including your arms and legs, can suffer from the elements as much as your face. It can be burned by the sun in the summer and can become very dry and flaky. This is particularly so in the winter months when you are in centrally heated rooms for most of the day. Even though moisture is water, it is not a good idea to lie in the bath for a long time, your skin can become 'waterlogged' (when it looks all crinky at the toes and fingertips). If this happens, you lose even more moisture through rapid evaporation. The best thing to do when you have stepped out of your bath or shower and dried yourself, is to rub body lotion all over while your skin is still warm and very slightly damp. If you have very dry elbows and knees, they will benefit from having the residue of your face cream rubbed into them. Your hands especially show the effects of ageing quite quickly so use hand cream whenever you can.

A good skin is something that most people can achieve given some care and attention.

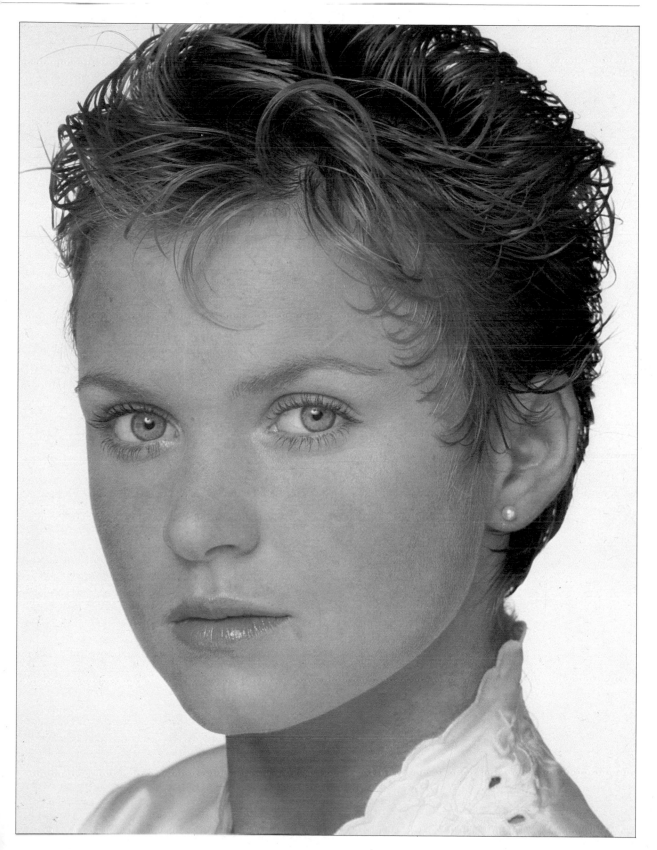

Routine

You are probably familiar with the classification of skin into dry, normal and oily types, but whatever category your skin falls into, it is likely to change with age. For instance, a spotty, greasy skin, which is troublesome at 15, may well be very dry by the time you reach 30. So you must reassess your skin type as you get older.

Once you have established your skin type, with the help of the chart, you can decide on the right way to care for it. Many women say they do not have time for a skin care routine but in fact it should be possible. There are not many things to do, and once it has become a habit, it will be as automatic as brushing your teeth.

Spasmodic skin care is next to useless, and will not produce results, whereas if you follow a regular programme, you will certainly reap the benefits. If you have time to chat on the telephone or talk with a friend over coffee you have time to take care of your complexion. You can even put all your items on a tray and carry out your routine in front of the television if you cannot drag yourself away from it!

Basically all skin types need to be kept clean and moist. There are three stages in this process – cleansing, toning and moisturising. The first stage is cleansing. Cleansers are available for all skin types, and in addition to removing make-up they will help to get rid of deep pore dirt. Eye make-up should be taken off with a product specially formulated for the job. If you like to use soap and water as well as a cleanser, that is fine, but not every type of soap is suitable. Always use non-perfumed soap and rinse your skin very well afterwards.

The next step, toning, removes any cleanser left behind and refreshes the skin. Although there are many products available for toning, you can use rosewater or ordinary water if it is suitable for your skin type. Bottled waters are good too, but not the fizzy type.

After toning, *always* moisturise. Even oily skins can lose water and become dry and flaky on the surface. Remember that moisture is water, not grease.

Whatever your skin type, always apply all creams and lotions to your skin with clean fingertips or cotton wool. Rather than using the cotton wool dry, damp it slightly so that it absorbs less of the product and more of it goes on your skin. Smooth the lotion or cream up and out over the forehead and cheeks, up the neck, down the nose and chin and gently inwards around the eyes, remembering that the area around the eyes is delicate. It does not have much muscle support and needs special care. In fact, never pull your skin about under any circumstances, even if you are giving your face a gentle massage.

A facial massage is wonderfully relaxing if done in a salon by a professional beautician. Although it is not quite so relaxing to massage your own face, it is certainly beneficial if you have a dry skin. The important things to remember are, firstly, to choose a fairly greasy cream, like a night cream or an oil such as almond, which will enable your fingers to slide across the skin without dragging it and, secondly, to keep all the movement going in an upward direction except for around the eyes, where you should pat very gently. A massage once a week is sufficient.

	DRY/SENSITIVE	NORMAL	OILY/ACNE
SKIN TYPES	Often looks 'thin' and feels 'tight' after cleansing, and will react by becoming red or blotchy if it is sensitive. It is prone to dry patches and flaking, and becomes lined when quite young.	This skin type, although it can have the odd spot, looks clear, and feels neither tight nor greasy after cleansing or washing. It *can* become dry if not looked after properly.	Oily skin looks and feels greasy soon after cleansing or washing. It is often accompanied by blackheads and/or spots and pimples. It has a tendency to look open pored and dull.
CLEANSING	Cream cleansers in a jar or a tin, or a very rich liquid are the most suitable for your skin type. If you want to wash you can use a superfatted non-perfumed soap, and rinse well.	Creamy liquid or cream cleansers are the best for your skin type. They can be marked normal to dry. Soap should be simple white soap or clear soap, non-perfumed.	Oily skin cleansers may be a lotion or a milk type. Acne skin cleansers are often medicated liquids. Soap or washing products are made especially for oily/acne skins, sometimes with oatmeal.
TONING	Pick a mild freshener (without alcohol), or use rosewater or cool water.	You can use a freshener (without alcohol), rosewater or non-fizzy mineral water.	Usually marked astringent, or suitable for acne skin (not for use around eyes or throat). Often special lotions or creams can be recommended by your doctor, some of which can be left on overnight.
MOISTURISING	Cream moisturisers in a jar.	Choose a thin cream or a thick lotion.	A very light non-greasy liquid is the most suitable for both these skin types.
TIPS	Read all labels carefully to make sure nothing contains alcohol. Look for the word 'hypo-allergenic' if you have a sensitive skin. Always use a moisturiser, night and day. The areas around your eyes may need a special eye cream. Give your face and throat a gentle massage with a rich cream once a week (especially in the winter).	Do not take it for granted — you must make an effort to keep it from becoming dry. Do not expose it to extremes of temperature. Watch out for products that are drying to the skin, like medicated soaps and cleansers. Apply moisturiser to a slightly damp face to help seal in the water.	See your doctor if acne develops. Keep your hands — except when cleansing — off your face and hair. Cleanse as often as necessary in between the morning and night routines. Do not use wash cloths or flannels on your face, and always dry with disposable paper towels. Never pick at spots, pimples, or blackheads.

SKIN SPECIALS

Creams

Very rich creams are available for lubricating dry skins. These can be massaged into your face and throat and left on for 20 minutes before blotting away the surplus with a tissue.

Special eye creams are useful for patting around the areas of the eye which, particularly in dry skins, are prone to fine lines.

All-purpose products, usually very thick white creams, are very useful for general skin care purposes for normal skin.

Almond, olive or Vitamin E oils are good for lubricating dry skin.

Medicated products

Usually only suitable for acne or disturbed skin and often recommended by doctors.

Clear lotion in tubes or bottles is available for drying up spots in specific areas.

Medicated foundations and cover-up sticks are available.

Washing products

Special soaps and washing agents are to be found for both oily/acne'd

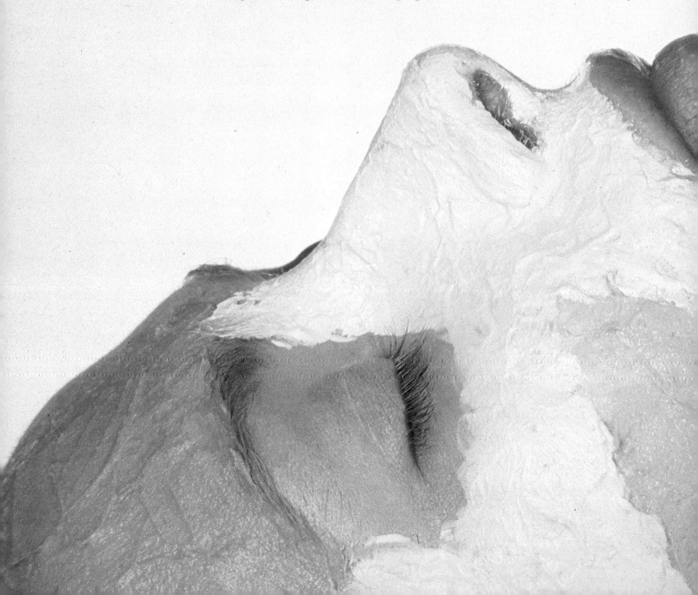

skins and for dry or delicate skins – *read the labels carefully*. They are really useful for people who do not feel 'clean' unless they have used water on their face.

Pore grains or products marked 'exfoliating' are good for deep cleansing and for sloughing off the tough or dead top layers of your skin. *Use with extreme care* and talk to the consultant when you buy, as to how often they are suitable for *your* skin.

Face masks
Every skin type benefits from regular use of a face mask. There are products available in many forms for *every* type of skin – again you can find out which one is for you by reading the label.

Use about once a week or more often if necessary (as in the case of oily skin which looks dull).

You can use different types of mask for different areas of your face and throat as needed – i.e. an oily skin mask on nose and chin and dry skin masks on cheeks, forehead and throat.

Only use in eye area if it says so on the pack.

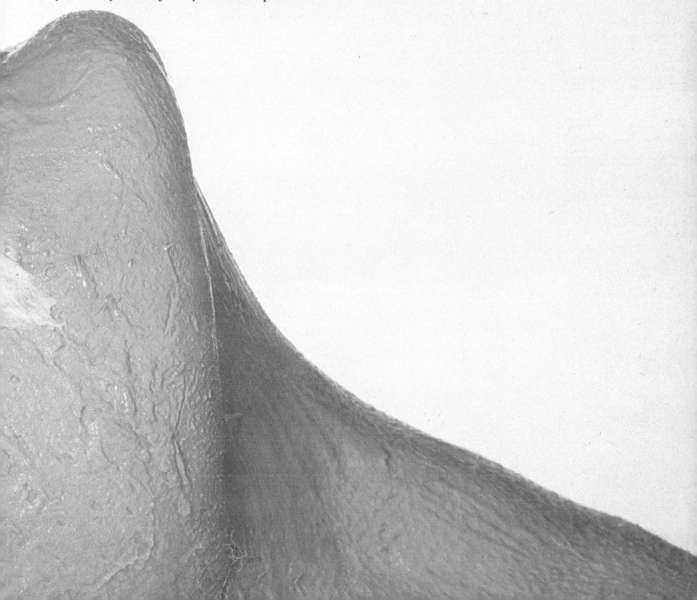

FOUNDATION

The first step after preparing your skin for make-up is to apply a coloured liquid or cream, which is called a foundation. Nearly every skin colour, type and texture can look better if the proper foundation is used. If your skin is really wonderful, or if you are very young, you may be lucky enough not to need a foundation at all.

The purpose of foundation is to make the skin look as smooth and clear as possible and to even out the colour. It forms a barrier between you and the elements and also provides a smooth base, which facilitates the application of other make-up on top – hence, the term base.

Choosing foundation

Contrary to popular belief foundation is not designed to give you a face which is an entirely different colour from your neck! Foundations come in a large variety of colours, textures and types, and vary a great deal in price. When you are buying a foundation, try to go to the store without any make-up on your skin. It is also a good idea to take a friend along with you to help you choose. Do not pick a colour just because you like the look of it in the bottle. Try to be realistic about the colour of your skin and to enlist your friend's help or ask the beauty consultant or sales-person (if they seem the sort of person you can talk to). Choose a colour, or colours, which you think might be right for you. You do this by matching it up to skin on your face and neck, *not* by trying it on the back of your hand, which usually bears no resemblance to the colour of your face and neck. Apply some to your face, then take your courage in both hands and go out of the shop into the daylight, taking your trusty friend with you (or alternatively your handbag mirror) and look at the colour of the foundation on your skin. If it stands out as a bright blob on your cheek, it is not the right colour! If it matches fairly well, you have probably got the right shade. You may find that your skin colour falls between two shades. In this case try mixing the two: a combination could be the answer. When combining colours, you can put a drop of each on the back of your hand and mix them up before applying them to your face. If you do buy two colours in bottles you could be very clever and decant them into another larger clean bottle. If they are packaged in other ways you will probably have to continue mixing them on the back of your hand, or with an applicator.

Once you have found the right colour foundation you must make sure you buy the right kind and texture for your skin type. You may find that you need different kinds of foundation depending on the time of year. For instance, in the summer, if you are lightly tanned and your skin looks really good, you may only need the lightest of gel make-ups to give you the look you want, whereas in the winter you may feel you need a heavier foundation to give you a smoother colour and also more protection from the weather. If your skin is good you may not want or need to put foundation all over your face at all, only on the patches which are prone to discolouration – for example, top of the cheeks, bridge of the nose and eyelids.

The kinds of foundation you will have to choose from are numerous and fall into specific categories. Medicated foundation is best suited to

Foundation – which is the basis of most good make-up – comes in many different textures and shades. The one that you choose depends on your own skin type and colour.

14

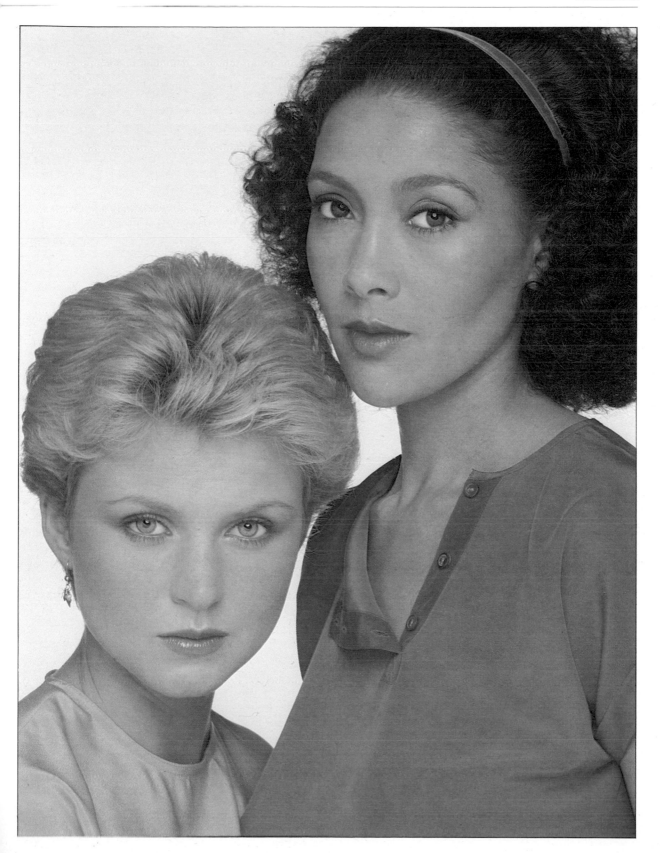

skins which tend to be spotty. There are special matt foundations with anti-shine for greasy skin which are useful for people in their teens and twenties. Liquids in bottles or tubes are the most popular types of foundation since they suit nearly every skin type and seem to work well for most women in their twenties and thirties. If you have a very dry skin you may find that a slightly richer cream in a pot, a stick-type make-up, or cake in a compact (which usually comes with its own sponge applicator) are the most suitable for your skin. This type is effective for women of over 40 who may have very dry skin. Foundations in a tube which say they combine both base and powder (called all-in-one make-up) can suit some skins, but they can be a bit drying. Gels are great for using in the summer when you only need a little coverage to match the tan on your face to that of your body, but they are quite difficult to apply evenly and must be put on with a clean sponge. Some foundations have a shine or glitter of some sort in them, but it is not a good idea to apply them all over your face, because they can make skin look very shiny and porous. Use them for highlighting as part of an evening make-up. Some foundations also include a sunscreen, which gives some protection to your skin from harmful ultra-violet light. A tinted moisturiser may double-up as a base on really good skin. Green-toned moisturiser or foundation is useful for toning down the redness on skins that have a very high colour.

Application

Most foundation can be applied with a slightly damp sponge (either a baby sponge or a cosmetic sponge). Damp does *not* mean wet, so squeeze the sponge out well in a towel or tissue. Very thin foundations are probably best applied with the finger tips as well as the sponge and you should certainly finish the blending of all foundations with your fingers.

Never apply foundation around the outer edges of your face since you will have nowhere to blend it into except your hairline. Do not forget to smooth it on *gently* around your eyes. If you have chosen the right colour it should not be necessary to apply it very far down your neck. Remember these points and you will avoid 'puddings' at the side of your face, and 'tide marks' around your neck!

If you have just smoothed moisturiser of any kind over your face and throat, remember to wait for five or ten minutes before applying your foundation, so that your skin has time to 'settle'. You should always give your moisturiser time to lose its stickiness.

It is a good idea to put moisturiser on immediately after you have washed in the morning. Then by the time you have had your breakfast and brushed your teeth, your face will be ready for make-up. If it is evening and you have just cleansed your face ready for a fresh application of make-up, follow the same procedure. (You can leave out the breakfast!)

You may find that after cleansing or bathing, your skin feels a bit warm or looks flushed. If you try to put on your make-up while your skin is not its normal colour, you may be tempted to apply more foundation than you need to cover the red areas.

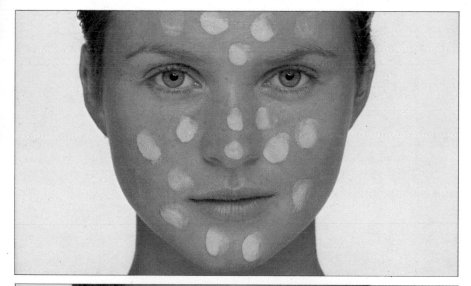

Dot the foundation all over the central area of your face.

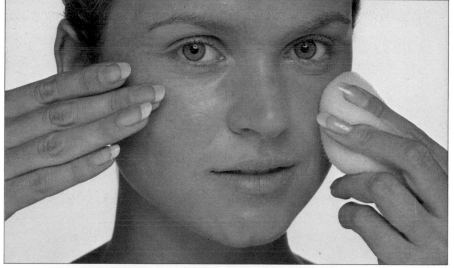

Blend it carefully with your applicator and smooth with your fingertips.

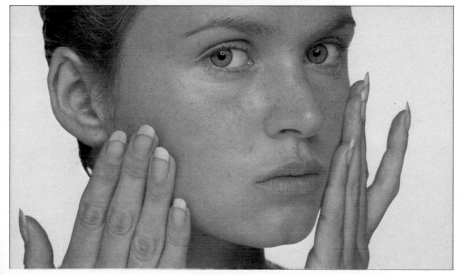

Check that it is even all over, and that you do not have hairline 'puddings' and 'tidemarks'. Do not forget the area just under your nose.

CONCEALER

Every face, no matter how young or how good the skin is, will have some marks or blemishes and will probably have dark shadows, particularly underneath the eyes. In addition there are often areas of discolouration to deal with, like redness across the nose and cheeks.

The best way to cover these is to use a heavier foundation in a light colour, or one of the concealing products specially made for the purpose. These can be bought in stick form (medicated or unmedicated), in a tube, or as a cream in a little pot. They sometimes have their own applicators. Dot the concealer in the required place with a fingertip or a little brush, and pat and press it on to the skin with your third finger. You can exert least pressure with that finger and will be less likely to drag delicate skin. Make sure that the colour is not too light, particularly round the eyes as you do not want to look like a startled panda! It should blend in well with your own skin tone. Use a little at a time as you can always add more later. If you do not wear foundation, you can use concealer by itself, wherever you need it.

(Top left) **Dot concealer carefully on shadows under the eyes, and on any marks or blemishes.**

(Top right) **Blend by patting and pressing onto your skin.**

(Bottom) **Make sure the final effect blends well with your skin tone, and that you do not have any 'pale' patches.**

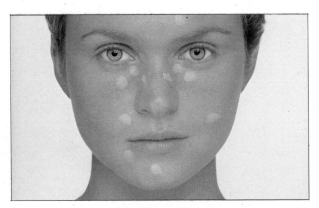

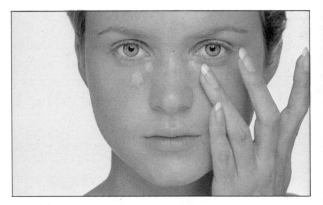

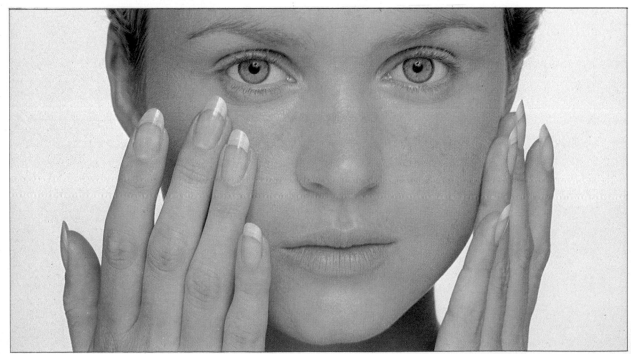

FACE FAULTS

There is no such thing as a perfect face, and certainly the idea of having a classic oval face is one that few people could aspire to. If you think your face is too long, round, squarc or pointed, do not worry about it.

Forget about drastic changes to the basic shape of your face, since this can only be done by clever shading, with great skill. If it is done badly you can look as if you have a dirty neck, five o'clock shadow or streaky cheeks. The shape of your face can be 'corrected' sufficiently by the skilful placing of blusher and anyway it is much better to emphasize all of the good points, than to try and disguise what only *you* regard as faults.

However, if you really have a very apparent face fault, it is possible to help minimize it by careful shading. Use a darker shade of foundation (avoid red tones) and make sure that you are standing in a really good light so that you can see what you are doing when you are making up.

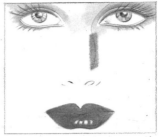

(Above) Dark foundation applied on the bumpy side of a crooked nose.

(Below) Carefully blended foundation to minimize a double chin.

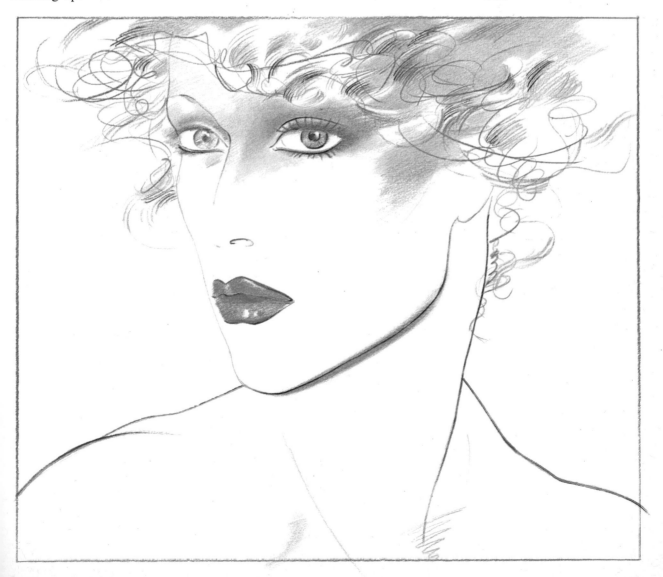

BLUSHER

Once you have understood how to use blusher correctly you will realise what a valuable cosmetic it can be. When used properly, it can enhance the face in a way that no other single product can. It can also add colour to the skin much more effectively than trying to enliven a pale face by putting on the wrong coloured foundation. However, many women worry about using blusher because they do not know what kind to use or where to apply it.

There are many different forms of blusher on the market, but basically they fall into three major categories: cream blushers, which come either in compacts, sticks or pencils; liquids, which can be either in a bottle or in a gel form in a tube; and the powder type. The last kind is perhaps the most popular type of blusher, particularly since it usually comes with its own applicator.

There is one rule to remember when applying any type of blusher – put on the liquid, cream or pencil types *before* you use face powder (if you are going to use it) and *after* moisturiser and/or foundation. Apply powder blushers *after* using face powder, or when the moisturiser and/or foundation have settled and your skin no longer feels sticky.

Applying blusher

Press your thumb just underneath your cheekbone, place your finger actually on the cheekbone, and imagine a teardrop shape on your cheek, with the rounded end nearest your nose, but no further in than the middle of your eyes. This is where you apply your blusher. Use your applicator, whether it be a sponge, brush or your fingers to blend the product in and make *really* sure that it does not have any hard edges. If the blusher is in the correct place it will automatically enhance the shape of your face. Never try to use it as a face shaper or you may look as though you have rusty coloured streaks down your cheeks. Make sure you keep blusher away from your hairline.

It is useful to have two or three shades of blusher – for instance, a brick tone, for wearing with all natural colours and browns; a soft red shade, for wearing with black and white or any of the really strong colours; and a soft pink which could be worn with all the blues, violets and pastels. Although this is a guideline to follow, you can wear any of the blushers with any colour clothes, as long as you apply them properly.

For the daytime, whether you use it on top of a foundation or if you have good skin which does not need foundation but does need colour, you may find that you like the look of liquid or cream blush on your face. It has a natural sheen which most powder blush does not have.

This makes it a very useful type of blush for young faces or for those who have quite dry skins. Creams and liquids will take a little bit of practice before you can use them to their best advantage, but they are well worth it.

Save the blushers which have gold, pearl or shine of some kind in them for the evening. You can sometimes use the very, very light coloured ones to highlight your cheek bones. The evening is also a good time to dot a little bit of blush on your temples and chin to give your face an extra glow. Do not use too much, though, because you will not want to look flushed.

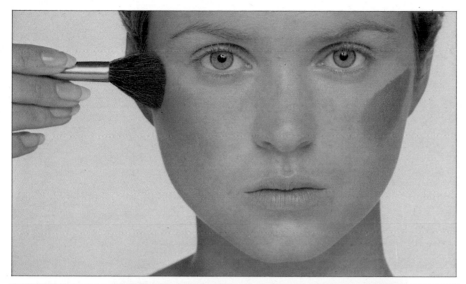

Apply powder blush with a brush after face powder. Apply cream or liquid blush with your fingertips before face powder.

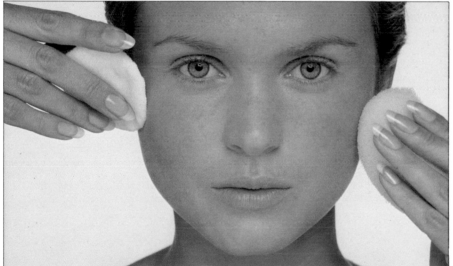

Soften the edges of powder blush with a puff. Blend cream or liquid blush with a sponge.

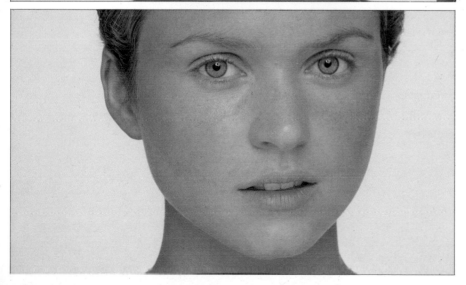

Make sure that the finished result has blended edges and no blotches.

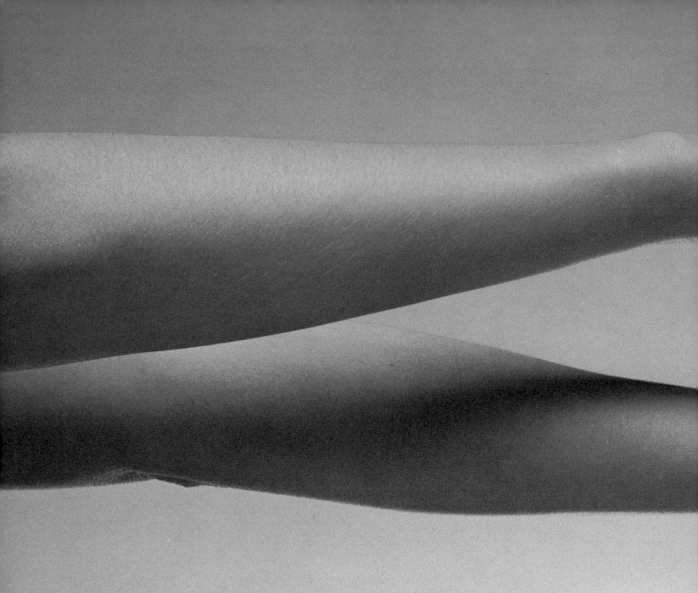

POWDER

Powder is a very underrated cosmetic. It really is the finishing touch to a good make-up, no matter how simple that make-up may be. It stops the face from looking shiny, without losing the natural sheen of the skin, and helps to set the make-up. It also helps to stop the 'creasing' of cosmetics such as cream eye shadows and eye pencils. Powder is available in many different forms and colours. Unless you have a very dark skin and can find a powder which is a good match to it, it is better to stick to one which is totally transparent or colourless. Transparency is not to be confused with translucency: 'translucent' is a term usually used to indicate that the powder is light in texture.

Face powder comes in two forms: loose, usually sold in a large round powder box; and compressed, which comes in a compact, and is usually sold with its own powder puff or brush applicator. Some face powders have pearl or glitter in them, but they are best reserved for use in the evening, and certainly are not intended to be used all over the face, as this can make your skin look very sweaty and greasy.

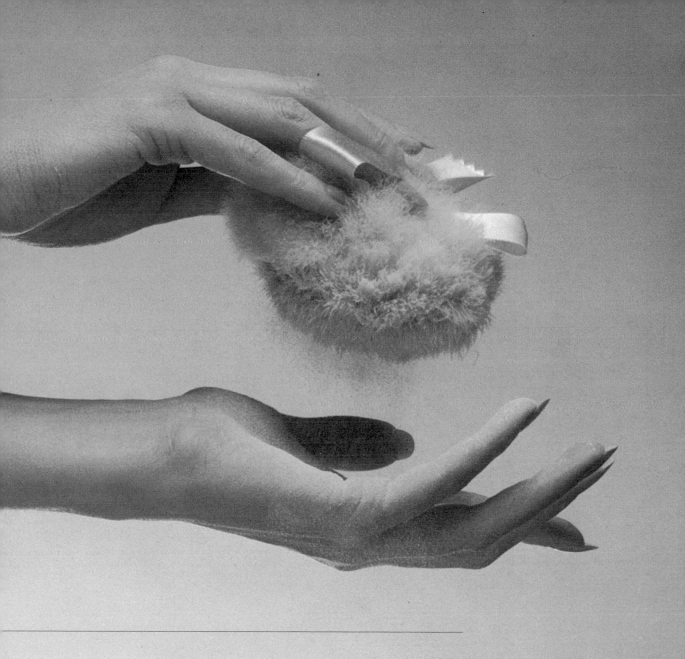

Never use a dirty applicator to apply your face powder, and never pick up a lot of powder on the applicator and put it straight on to your face. Always knock off the excess powder on to the palm or the back of your hand, before applying.

Loose powder is good to use on most occasions, but compressed powder is perhaps easier to carry around for touching up. You can use compressed powder all the time if you find that it suits you. Remember that even transparent face powder will slightly alter the colour of any make-up underneath it by lightening it just a little. Use face powder before you use *any* powder cosmetics, i.e. powder blushers, powder eye shadows, etc, but *after* you have used cream or pencil cosmetics, such as cream blush or eye-shadow sticks.

Concentrate on using most of the powder in the central areas of your face, and the smallest amount over the cheekbones and around your eyes. This avoids it settling into fine lines around your eyes, or getting caught up in the downy hairs at the sides of your face.

LOOSE POWDER

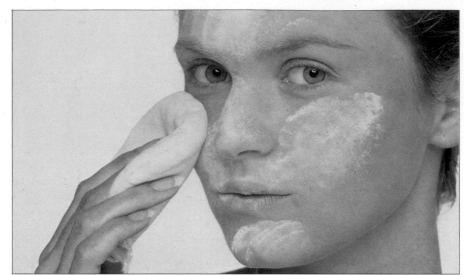

Apply loose powder by slapping and pressing it firmly into the foundation, without rubbing.

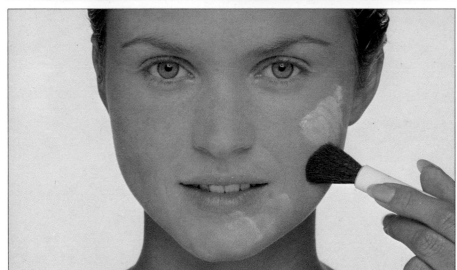

Gently dust off the excess using a puff or brush. Take care to powder around the nostrils and chin.

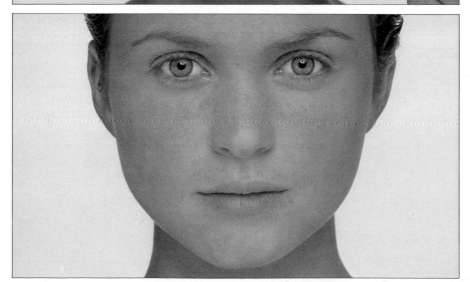

Check that powder is well blended over the face, and that there are no shiny or powdery patches.

COMPRESSED POWDER

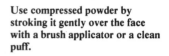

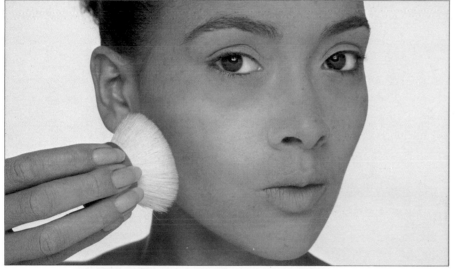

Use compressed powder by stroking it gently over the face with a brush applicator or a clean puff.

Blend by continuing the same movements all over the face, taking care not to rub the skin.

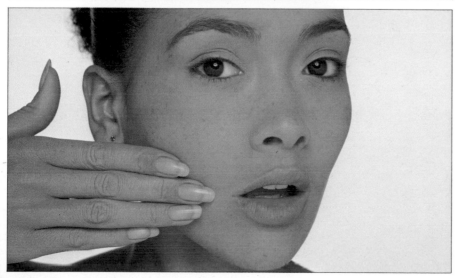

Inspect the finished result carefully to make sure that it does not look uneven or 'caked' in any one spot, especially the nose and chin area.

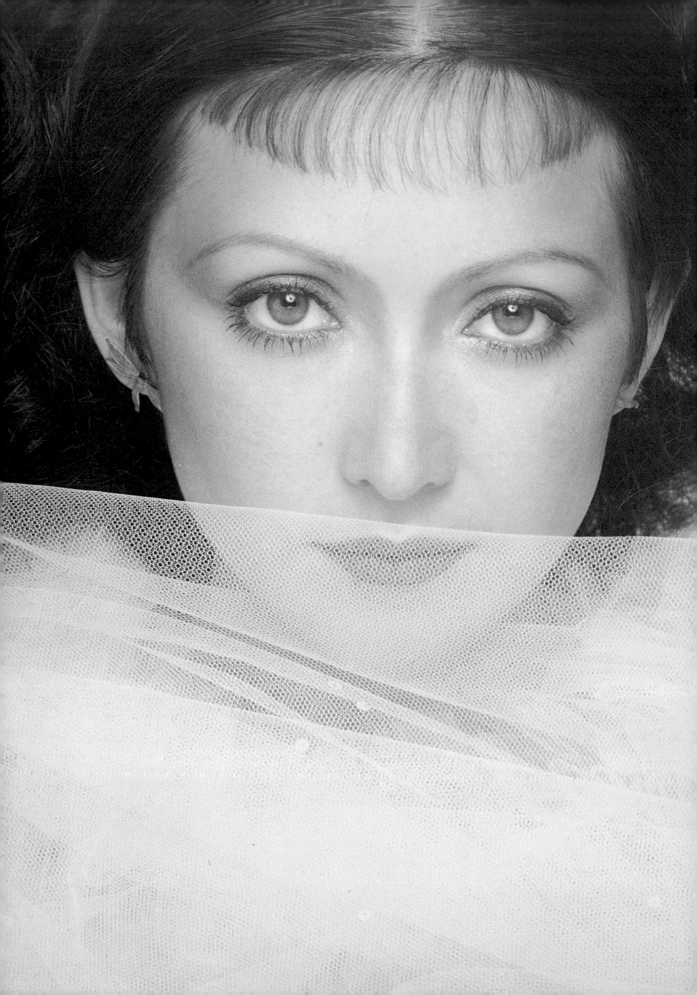

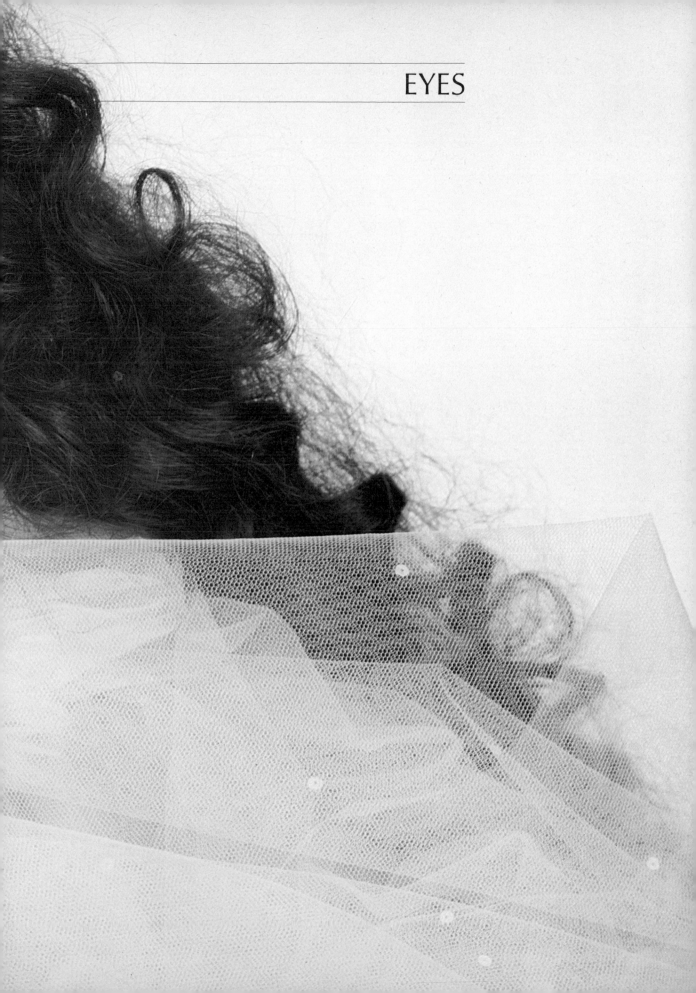

EYES

Whenever you talk to someone, you tend to look at their eyes. The eyes are very expressive, they reflect emotion without the use of the spoken word. They are also a good indication of your general state of health. After all, one of the first parts of the body that your doctor checks is your eyes. Eye make-up can be a very simple affair, or it can be a marvellous artistic creation. It has its roots in ancient cultures of all kinds, and is often used as an important part of mime, theatre and dance. But for most people it would be sufficient to be able to make up their eyes beautifully. If you use a little bit of imagination and you master the basic techniques of how to choose and how to apply your eye make-up, you will find you can create the kind of eyes that you always see on models in magazines.

A choice of products

Just being able to choose the right kind and colour of eye make-up may seem to be an insurmountable task when you see the enormous variety available on most cosmetics counters. Your first thought is sure to be, 'Where do I begin?' To start with then, a definition of what all these products are:

Eye-shadow colour comes in many forms, ranging from pots of cream eye-shadow and compressed eye shadow, through to plain or sparkly eye shadow in plastic tubes with the applicator attached to the lid. There is a huge variety of thick and thin, frosted and unfrosted *eye pencils* which can be used as eye colour, eyeliner, as eyebrow pencils

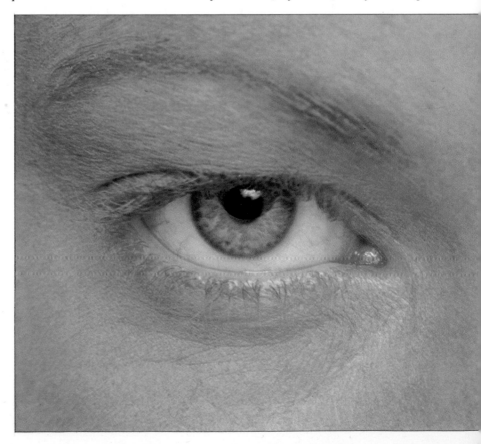

or as kohl to be put on the inside edge of the bottom eyelid. *Eyeliners*, for defining the eye, usually comes in two forms, as a pencil, or as a cake, which you wet and apply with a fine brush. The final touch to eye make-up is *mascara*. One form comes in a wand with a spiral brush applicator, and sometimes with a comb. This kind can have added fibres to make your lashes look longer, and can be waterproof. The other type of mascara available is the cake type, which is usually found in a small compact and has to be put on with a mascara brush. However, it should not be applied in one thick coat. It is much better, and far more effective, to keep the lashes separate by applying two or three thin coats. Mascara can be worn by itself or in conjunction with other make-up. It is very important to make sure that you remove *all* eye make-up at the end of the day. Both kohl and mascara have a tendency to cling to the lashes, so make sure that they are properly cleaned off.

Colours

There are lots of misconceptions about what colour eye–shadow you should wear. It is not really true that if you have blue eyes you should only wear blue eye–shadow, or grey shadow if you have grey eyes. Anyway everyone thinks that their eyes are just one colour. We always refer to someone as having brown eyes or blue eyes, or whatever colour they may be. If we were to be more observant, we would be more accurate if we described the eyes as being composed of several

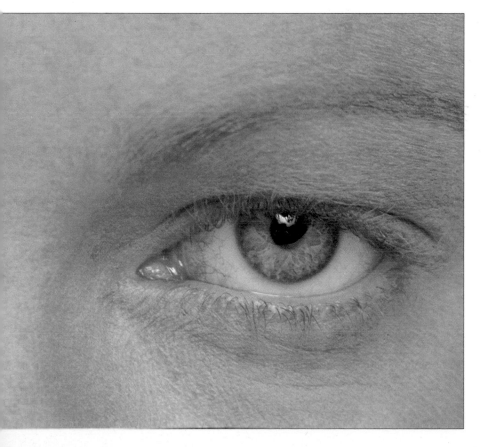

One of the most common of eye shapes is one where the eyes are deep set or do not have a lot of lid visible.

colours. Unless you have very dark brown eyes you can see this for yourself by just looking closely at your own eyes in a mirror. The colours you see on the iris could be a very good guide to what colours to choose when you are buying eye make-up. For instance blue eyes could have flecks of grey, amber, green, dark blue and sometimes even violet in them. A shade which matches the overall colour of your eye does not necessarily enhance the natural hue.

Very pale chalky colours, such as pale blue and pale green can make the eyes look small. These colours are very hard and look unnatural especially in daylight. But they are perfect for use as highlighters. If you have enough eyelid showing, you can use a little highlighter in a soft tone which matches your eyelid colour on the centre of your lid, but mostly it is best used to emphasize the brow bone. This is the area directly below the eyebrow.

It is so easy to get stuck in an eye make-up rut and still be wearing the same type of eye make-up and colour of eye–shadow as you were five or ten years ago. Although you probably pay attention to changing fashions and seasons, you must also take into consideration the fact that your age changes too. You change your hair and style of dress over the years, so why should your eye make-up stay the same?

A good basic rule to bear in mind when you are going to buy eye make-up is to leave the bright, strong, or very shiny eye colours for use after dark. Stick to the muted soft colours like sludgy greens, greys and browns for day, since they are much more flattering and easier to

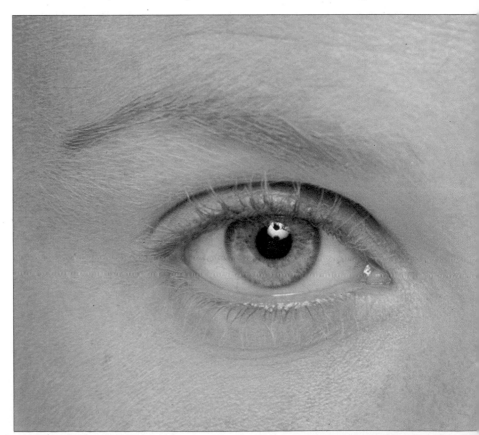

wear. If your eyelids are particularly crêpey, you really should avoid eye–shadows which are shiny or pearly as this just emphasizes the 'elephant hide' effect! If you remember that all cream or pencil eye–shadows should be applied before face powder, and that the powder eye–shadows can be put on after powdering, you will avoid having messy looking make-up.

Lots of eye–shadows come with their own applicators or brush, but it is a good idea, in any case, to buy some make-up brushes. You can get these in most department stores, or you can buy two or three soft chisel-ended paint brushes in an art shop. They are invaluable for blending away hard edges and giving your make-up a really professional finish. It is important to remember to keep all your eye products clean and in good condition, so as to avoid the risk of eye infections. This of course applies to everything you use on your face. Something you think may be an allergy could well be caused by the use of a less than clean applicator.

Eyelash curlers, once you have mastered the trick of using them, are very good for making the eyes look really open and bright. Remember however not to pull them away from your eyes without opening the 'scissors' fully first.

Beautiful eyes are best achieved by good health, the right amount of sleep, and avoidance, as far as possible, of smoky atmospheres and a lot of alcohol (this goes for your skin too). No amount of eye make-up will make your eyes sparkle if they are puffy and bloodshot!

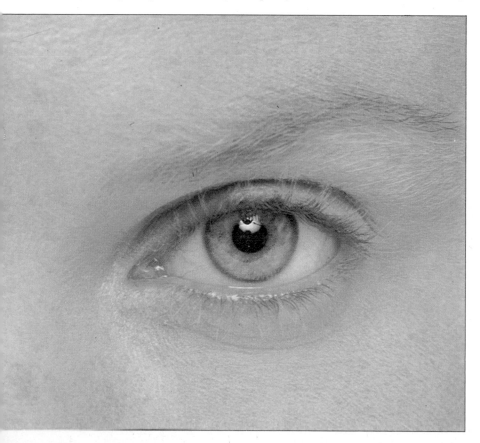

The other common eye shape is one where the eye has an average amount of lid showing or droops slightly at the outer corner.

DEEP-SET EYES

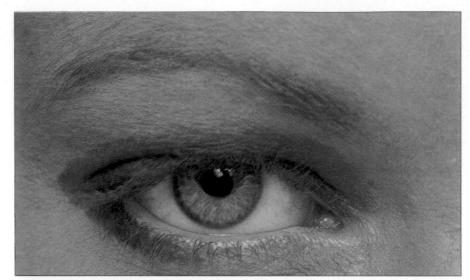

Put your chosen colour all over the top lid, and a little halfway down the bottom lid.

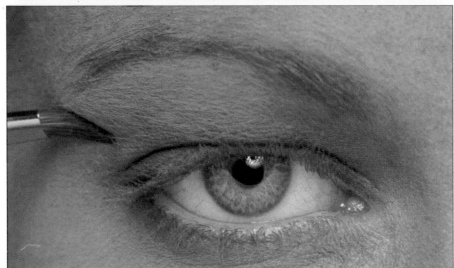

Blend the colour carefully up towards the brow and soften the edges on the lower lid with a brush.

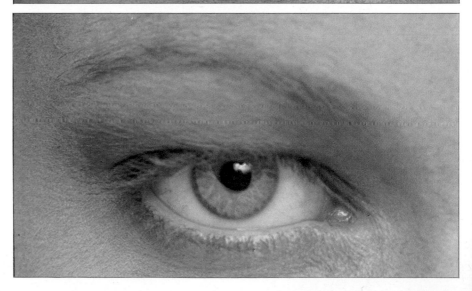

Check that the shadow is well blended everywhere.

LIDDED EYES

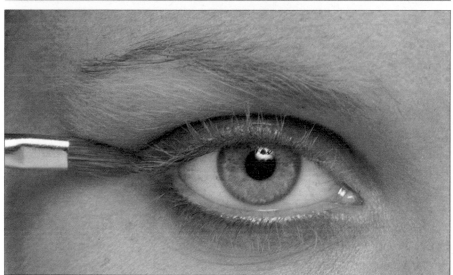

Apply the shadow colour in the socket line and in a 'V' shape in the outer edges of the eye.

Fade away all the hard edges of the shadow on the upper and lower lids with a brush.

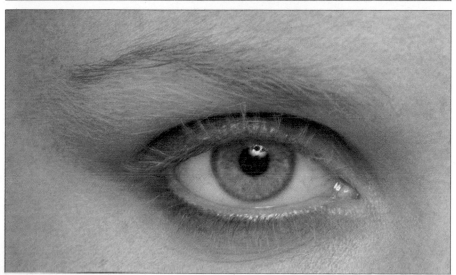

Make sure that the shading on both eyes is equal before continuing.

EYELINER

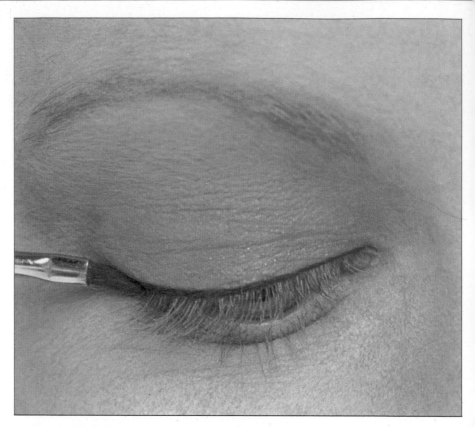

Paint on a narrow line of eyeliner as close as possible to the top lashes. No big 'ticks' at the corner!

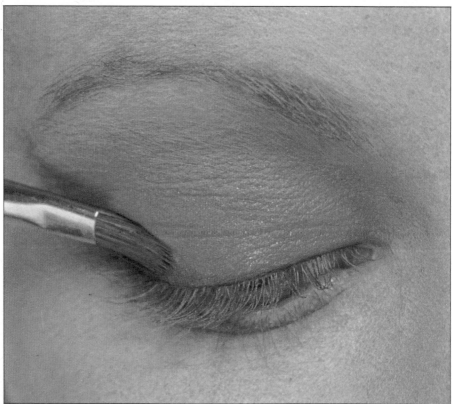

Use a slightly damp brush to stroke over the hard edge of the eye line blending it into the eye-shadow.

KOHL

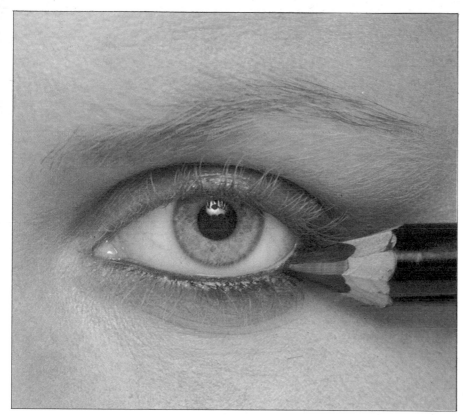

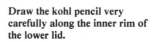

Draw the kohl pencil very
carefully along the inner rim of
the lower lid.

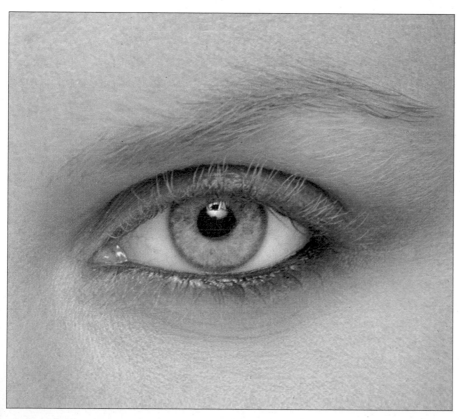

Make sure that the kohl colour
blends properly into the lower lid
colour (if used) and that it has not
'collected' in the eye corner.

HIGHLIGHTER

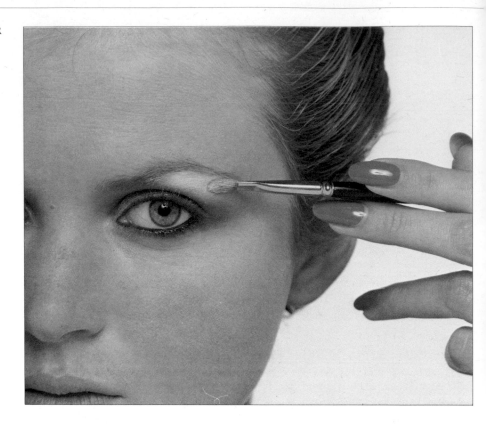

Stroke the highlighter carefully
along the brow bone.

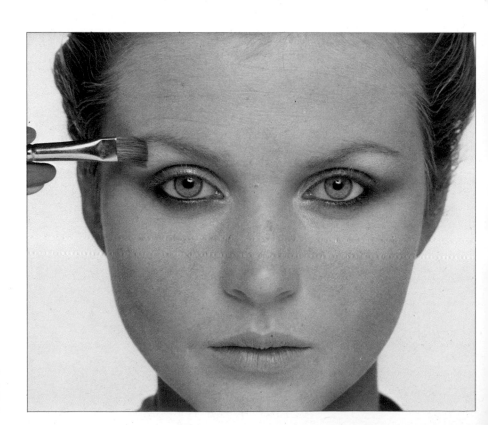

Use a clean brush to blend the
highlighter so that it looks like a
soft sheen rather than a hard
shine.

MASCARA

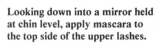

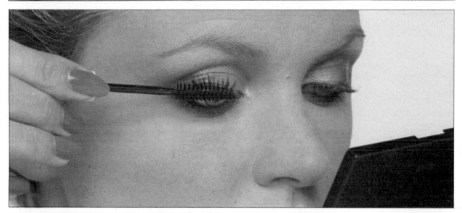

Looking down into a mirror held at chin level, apply mascara to the top side of the upper lashes.

Keeping the mirror at chin level, put mascara on the underneath of the top lashes.

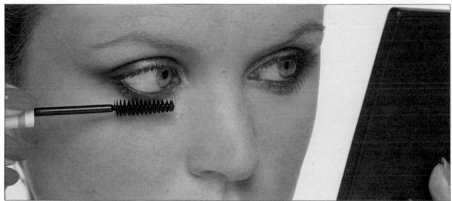

Hold the mirror up and keep your chin down to mascara the lower lashes.

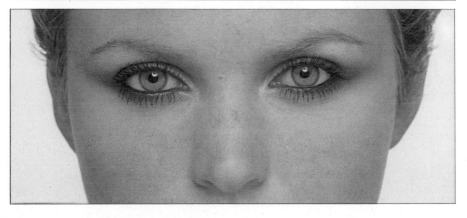

Check that your lashes are not stuck together and that the inner and outer corners have been covered.

LIPS

Every so often it either becomes fashionable or unfashionable to emphasize your mouth. For hundreds of years women (and men) have shaped and coloured their lips. The mouth is alleged to indicate the type of person you are. For instance we often say that people who have very thin lips are bound to be mean. Obviously this does not hold true, but there is no doubt that a well balanced lip shape that tends to tilt up at the corners, rather than down, definitely gives the face a nicer expression. Fashion in lip colour seems to swing from nearly black to practically flesh-toned and back again, depending on which part of the face (eyes or lips) is the focus of attention at the time, and is being emphasized.

Lipsticks

Lipstick is the final touch to the make-up and can really make the face come alive. Many women who never wear any other cosmetic, wear lipstick. It comes in a variety of containers, which do not always indicate the type of product that is likely to be found inside.

Conventional *stick lipsticks* can either give good coverage or can be a very thin gloss. Lipsticks also come in *compacts*, sometimes with a brush, and can vary in density as can those in the conventional stick form. You can also find lipstick, or *lip gloss* in long tubes with their own applicator, or in little round pots. *Lip pencils* come in two thicknesses, thin for outlining the lips and thick for filling in.

Many lip colours can be bought with frosting of some kind, but remember that, although you may want to keep your lipstick light in texture and in tone, it is as well to avoid the very pale, pearlized lipsticks, since they only make the mouth look lined and dry. They are also very unflattering to the teeth, skin and eyes.

Lip colours

The choice of lip colours is huge, and although most people have their favourites, it is a good idea to have a little 'wardrobe' of colours and types. For instance, you could have one soft pinky-brown lip pencil and tinted lip gloss, for making the 'natural' type of mouth; a browny russet colour, either stick or compact, which would go with all the warm–coloured clothes you might wear; a muted raspberry shade which would suit every colour from navy blue to lavender and a soft red for wearing with black and white and any strong primary colours. Red also looks good when worn with very little other make-up, if your skin is in good condition, or if you have a light tan. Last but not least have a clear gloss to add shine to any of the above, or to wear just on its own.

If you feel that you really would like to try to alter the shape of your lips a little, there are a few things that you can do to deal with common faults. If your top lip appears to be too thin, use a pencil the same colour as your lips to draw just slightly over your natural line and then fill in with your favourite lipstick. However, if you think your bottom lip is not full enough fill it in with a shade or two lighter than you have used on your top lip. Should an over-full mouth be your problem, centre the colour and blend away to the edges.

Lipstick adds the final touch to a good make-up, or used on its own can make the face come alive.

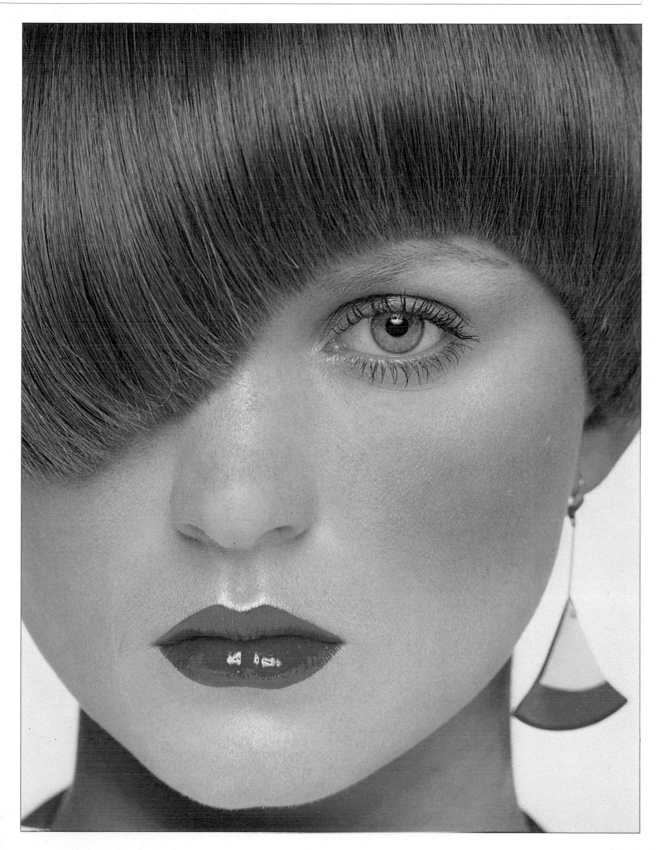

OUTLINING

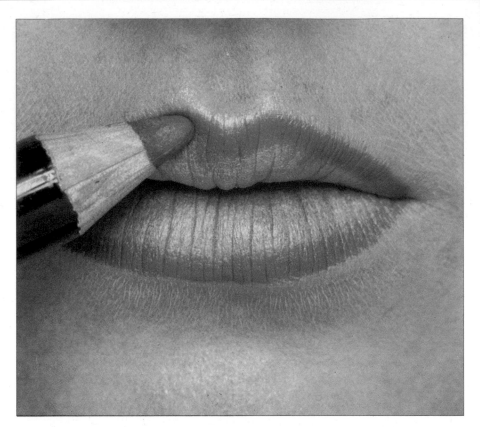

Outlining can be done with a pencil or lip brush. When using a pencil, sharpen it and draw an outline around your lips. Make sure that the colour tones with your chosen lipstick.

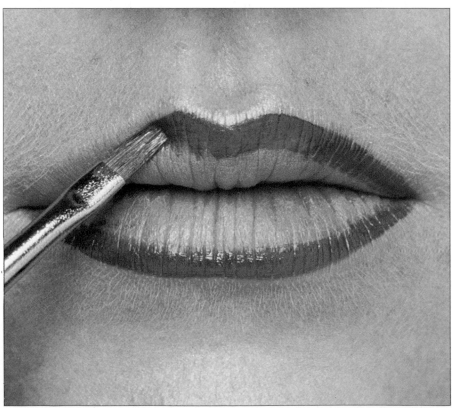

When using a lip brush rest your curled fingers on your chin to help steady your hand.

FILLING IN

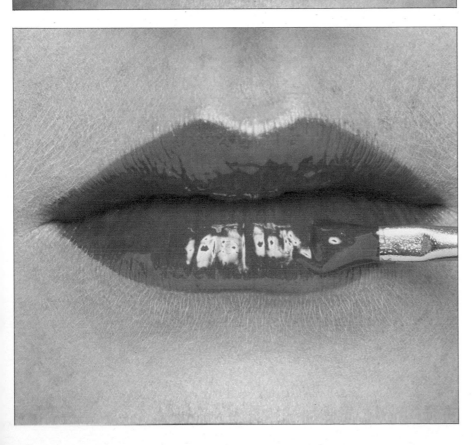

Fill in your lip colour either directly from a lipstick, or by using a lip brush.

Apply lip gloss very carefully and do not take it right to the edges of the mouth. This can cause the lipstick to run.

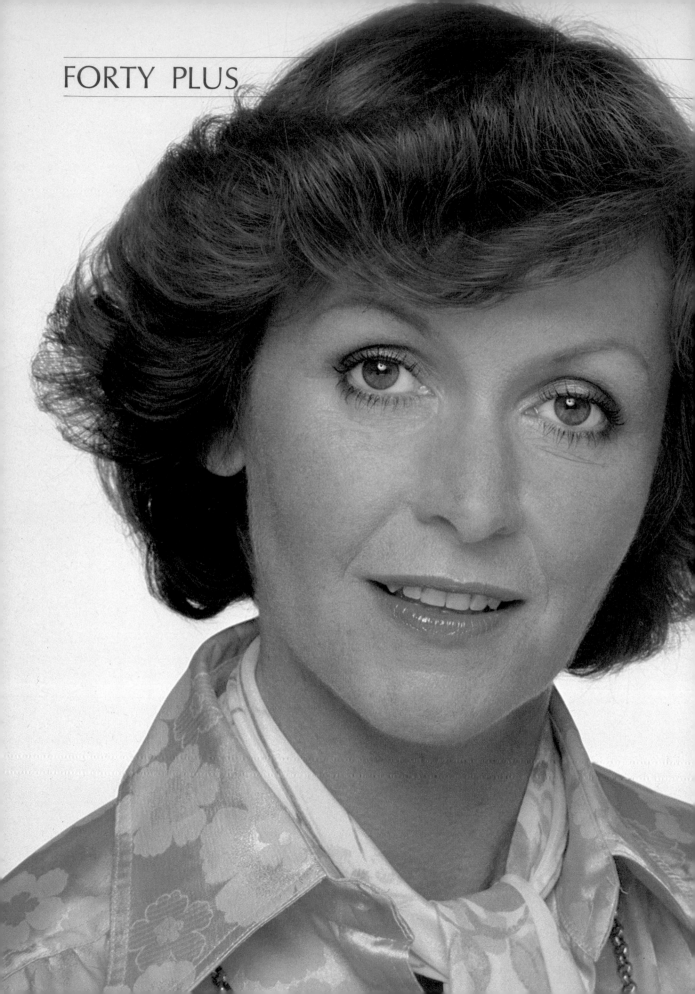

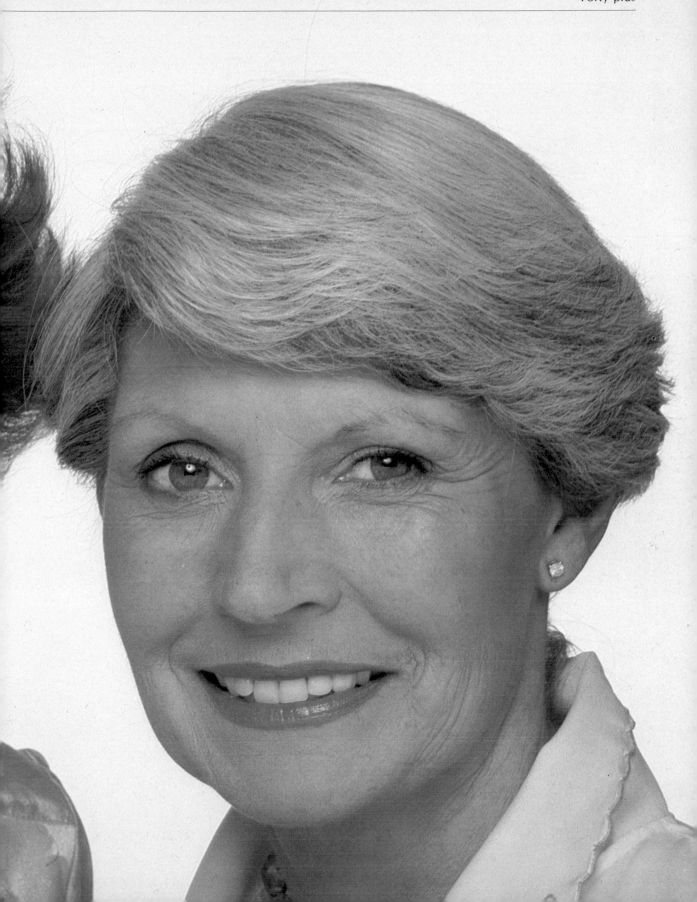

It is said that life begins at 40 and indeed it can. It used to be thought of as not the done thing for ladies of 40 and over to be taking a youthful interest in their face and body. Looking after your skin and keeping your figure in good shape was considered to be the prerogative of those much younger, and if you took an interest in your appearance and wore make-up, you were certain to be regarded as 'mutton dressed as lamb'. Even now if you are a woman over 25 and having your first pregnancy it comes as something of a shock to see yourself referred to on hospital notes as a mature mother! Happily, mature mothers of over 25, over 35 and sometimes over 45, can now look as good as they feel. So if you are 40 or over, you can start to reassess your appearance.

Many of them will find that they have more time to themselves and more energy to spare in their forties and that this is the time to think about what cosmetics to use, and how to use them. Perhaps *you* have spent the last 10 or 15 years working hard and bringing up a family and have got out of the habit of thinking much about your make-up.

First take a long hard look at yourself. Take off all your make-up -and go and stand in good clear daylight and try to be really honest about what you see in the mirror (you can be alone when you do this!) and own up to the fact that you have a few wrinkles by now. They probably cannot be erased but they can certainly be minimized. Now is the time to delay further ageing by looking afresh at your skin care

Dot on a soft cream or liquid blush with the fingertips. Use a slightly damp sponge to blend the blush well into the foundation so that it looks soft and smooth.

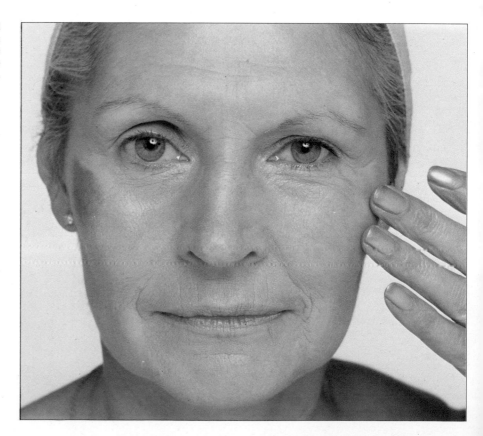

routine and making sure that you really stick to it. Even if you had very oily skin when you were young, it is quite likely now that this condition has evened out somewhat. You probably do not have very many spots or pimples and you will find that your skin is a lot less lined than that of your friends who have dry skins. So there is a silver lining to every 'spotty' cloud!

Skin aids

If your skin is drier than it used to be you will find that you need a richer moisturizer and a night cream. The richer moisturizers are usually to be found in cream form. Night creams do not necessarily mean that you have to go to bed with your face looking as though it has been painted with melted butter. To soften the lines round the eyes, it is a good idea to buy a special eye cream.

Face masks are invaluable, and using one at least once a week is both relaxing and beneficial. Unless your skin is very oily, do avoid ones which dry hard on the skin. Look for the packs marked 'for dry skin'. Apart from masks, do not forget to treat your throat and hands in the same way as you treat your face.

Your neck can become a much neglected area and sometimes, although the skin on your face is quite supple, the skin on your throat can look very parched and more deeply lined than your face. Quite often your posture can deepen the wrinkles on your face and you can

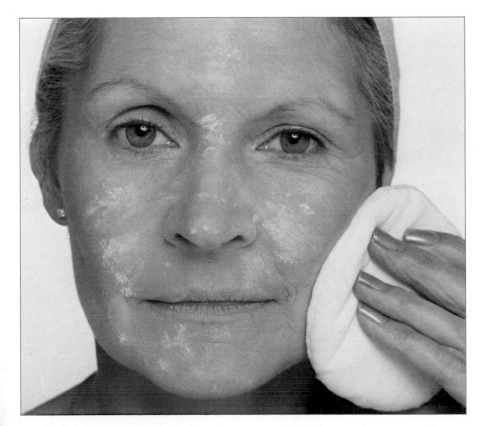

Pat loose powder on to the base, concentrating on the central area of the face, putting only the barest minimum around the eyes and on the cheeks. Make sure that none of the powder is 'settling' around the nostrils and that it is not emphasizing any fine lines around the eyes.

check this out for yourself. Stand in front of a mirror and imagine that there is a piece of string running up your spine and out of the top of your head. Align yourself with it by straightening your back and holding your head erect. The lines on your neck should lessen considerably.

Once you have corrected the wrinkles that are due to bad posture, you can discourage others from deepening by frequently applying skin cream. If you have dry skin on your hands, even though you regularly use hand cream, give them a treat two nights a week. Rub a rich skin cream and/or some almond oil into your hands and sleep wearing a pair of white cotton gloves.

You may find that you develop brown marks or 'liver spots' on your skin, as you grow older. These are the results of a build-up of pigment under the skin. There are products on the market which, if used over a period of time, can result in the gradual fading out of these marks. One word of caution, however, if you do use one of these treatment creams, take care to read thoroughly the leaflets provided and follow the instructions carefully. Also, if you try one of these products, do not forget that the marks can reappear or be made darker by exposure to the sun.

Foundation

After the age of 40 it is almost certainly better to totally re-think your make-up, and you will probably decide to keep it very subtle. Do not be drawn into thinking you have to use a dark foundation because you feel that your skin lacks colour. If you use eye make-up and blusher correctly, you will not look washed out.

Depending on just how dry your skin is, choose your foundation accordingly. Use a light rich liquid in a bottle or tube, or a cream. Take care when applying either because you need good coverage but you do not want to emphasize wrinkles. One of the best ways of putting just a very thin film of colour over the skin is to apply it with a barely damp sponge. This also stops you pulling the skin about too much.

Face powder is certainly good to use. Buy the totally colourless type and be very careful not to put very much around the eye area, since that will emphasize fine lines. Cream or liquid blusher leaves a more moist finish than a powder blusher. Make sure that you blend it in well at the edges and that you have not put on too much.

Eyes and lips

If the skin around your eyes is fairly smooth, you could choose almost any eye colour with the exception of frosted colour or quick-drying eye–shadows, as these emphasize wrinkles. Keep your colour choice subtle and neutral – soft greys, browns, very sludgy greens. When using eye colour do not put too much under the eyes because it often smudges downwards; just a little at the outer edges of the bottom lid is usually sufficient. Also, pick non-run mascaras. Leave the heavy black kohl pencils to younger faces and do not use black mascara, unless of course you are naturally very dark.

One of the big problems to deal with are the tiny lines that appear

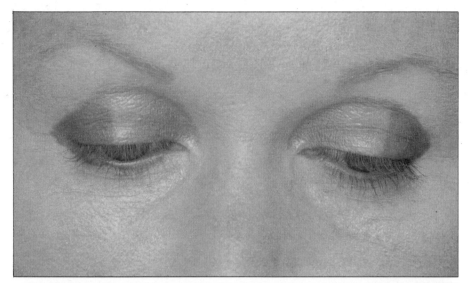

Apply one eye-shadow colour to the first two-thirds of the upper lid, and a darker shade to the last third of the lid. Take a little of it around the outer edge of the lower lid.

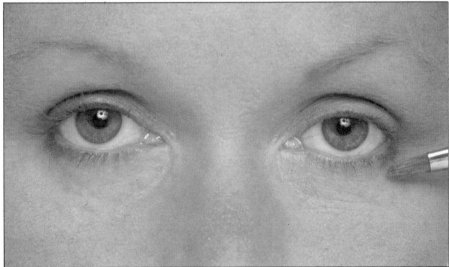

Use a soft brush to fade away any hard edges and to make the two colours blend into each other.

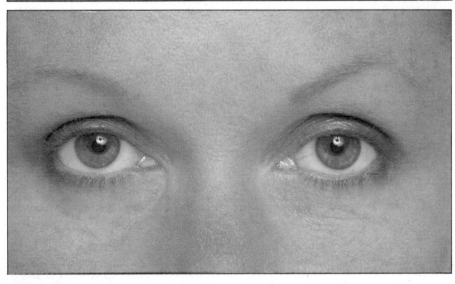

Check that the make-up is well blended, that there are no blotches and that both eyes are the same before adding mascara.

around the edges of the mouth. After a very short time, lipstick can smudge into these small lines and appear to be 'bleeding'. Although it is impossible to stop this happening completely you can certainly do something to help. Outline your lips carefully, using a lip brush or pencil. Blot the outline well on a tissue, then, keeping your lips together, smile, and pat the edges of your mouth very lightly with a little powder on your powder puff. This will help to stop it 'bleeding'. Then fill in with colour, but do not go right up to the edge of the mouth, and blot again very lightly.

(Top left) Draw the outline carefully with a lipbrush.
(Top right) Blot the outline well on a tissue.

(Bottom left) Smile, with your lips together, and lightly powder the edges of your mouth to prevent 'bleeding'.

(Bottom right) Fill in the lips with colour before blotting again, taking care not to go over the powdered edges, but making sure that the colours blend into each other.

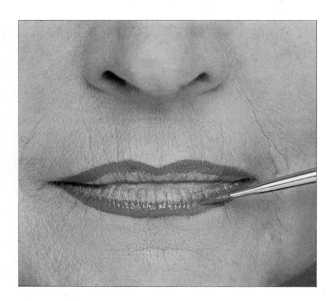

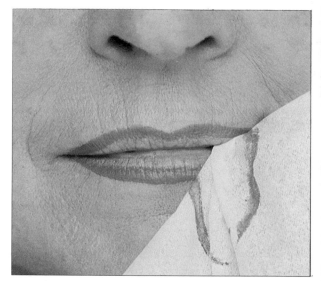

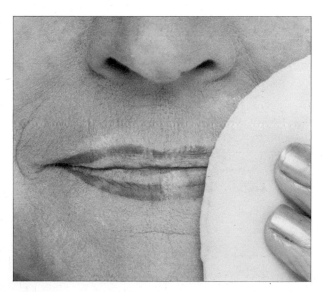

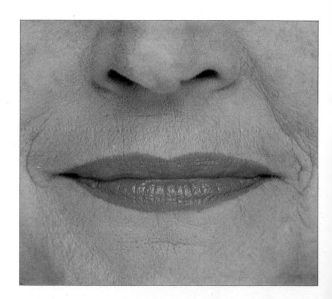

There are many cosmetics on the market which, although they can be used during the day, are probably best reserved for use after dark, since most of them are either very bright or contain frosting or glitter. Most of these cosmetics are products intended for use around the eyes. They come in every form of eye make-up from regular palettes of powder eye-shadow, right through to soft frosted pencils. There are even brightly coloured mascaras in green, blue and sometimes violet, which can look marvellous when used in conjunction with a matching eye-shadow. Unfortunately these coloured mascaras are only really effective if your lashes are quite fair. If you decide to use gold or silver glitter – a word of warning, be careful how you apply it, you only need a little and do not let the glitter anywhere near the rest of your make-up. It seems to cling to everything.

After-dark colours
The evening is a good time to experiment and you can risk using things that would look outrageous in the cold light of day. It is the time to try out colours you have always admired on other people and wanted to experiment with yourself. If you are in need of a little inspiration, take a careful look at how they are used in magazine photographs.

You can break the rule about foundation colour at night, and if you want to make your skin lighter or darker, now is the time to do it. But do reserve the foundations with glitter or frosting in them for use on cheekbones and do not put them all over your face – they will just make you look hot. The same applies to face powder with sparkle in it. Body glitter which usually comes in a gel or cream, is a great way of highlighting your shoulders or bare legs, or any other bit of you that you think is worthy of extra attention!

Matching make-up with clothes
In the evening you can use the really bright luminous eye-shadows, the ones with lots of shine in, and the gold and silver shades. You can use two or three together for maximum effect. If you are not sure just what colours to choose, try using your dress or jewellery as a guide, and wear colours to match. The same applies to the really vivid lip colours. You can often find a red or bright pink which matches very well with your outfit. Do use gloss on your mouth, but not too much, as you will probably be eating and drinking and you do not want it to smear. If you have nice hands, gold, silver or sparkly nail polishes will emphasize them. Again you can use more than one colour, perhaps red nails with sparkly gold tips – use your imagination!

Last but not least are false eyelashes. They too come into their own in the evening, but if you do not want to look as if you are wearing them, try fixing to the upper lashes, the fine lashes that are intended for the bottom lid. They thicken and lengthen the eyelashes without looking too obvious.

The best way to get the most out of your evening make-up is to look at what other people are doing, to really use your imagination, and above all feel beautiful and enjoy yourself!

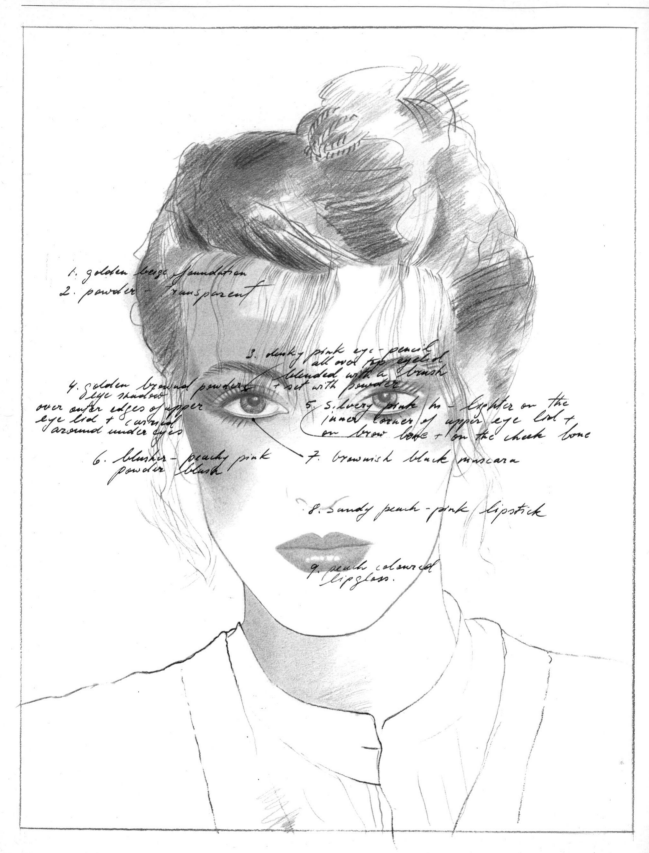

1. golden beige foundation
2. powder - transparent

3. dusky pink eye-pencil all over top eyelid blended with a brush + set with powder

4. golden brownal powder / eye shadow over outer edges of upper eye lid + carried around under eyes

5. silvery pink hi - lighter on the inner corner of upper eye lid + on brow bone + on the cheek bone

6. blusher - peachy pink powder /blush

7. brownish black mascara

8. sandy peach-pink lipstick

9. peach coloured lipgloss.

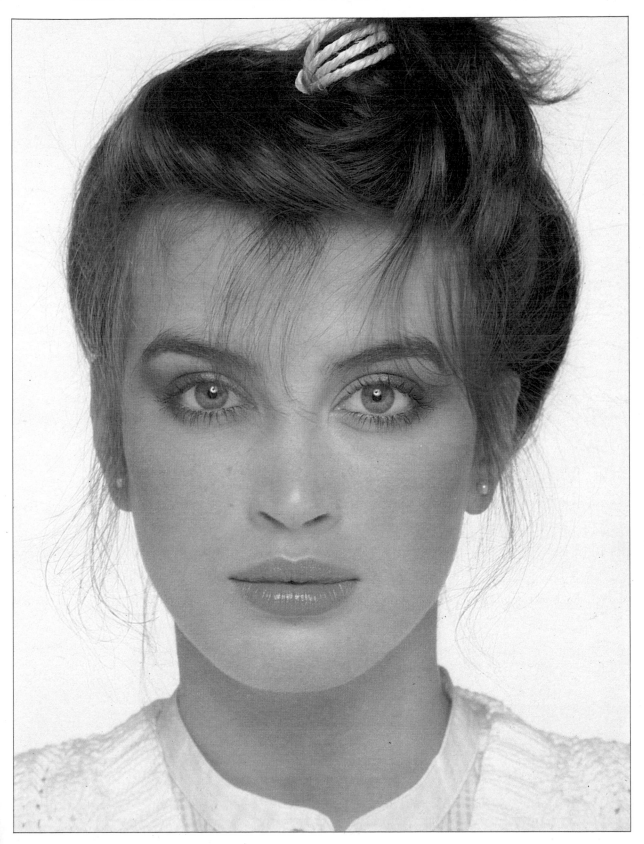

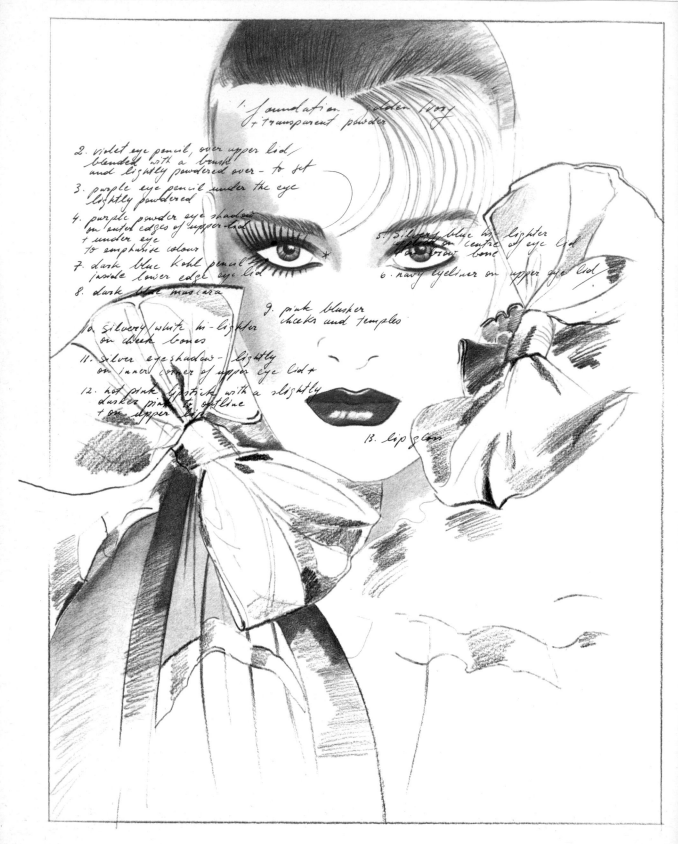

1. foundation – golden ivory
   + transparent powder

2. violet eye pencil, over upper lid,
   blended with a brush
   and lightly powdered over – to set

3. purple eye pencil under the eye
   lightly powdered

4. purple powder eye shadow
   on outer edges of upper lid
   + under eye
   to emphasise colour

5. silvery blue hi-lighter
   applied on centre of eye lid
   + on brow bone

6. navy eyeliner on upper eye lid

7. dark blue kohl pencil
   inside lower edge eye lid

8. dark blue mascara

9. pink blusher
   cheeks and temples

10. silvery/white hi-lighter
    on cheek bones

11. silver eyeshadow – lightly
    on inner corner of upper eye lid

12. hot pink lipstick with a slightly
    duskier pink to outline
    + on upper lip

13. lip gloss

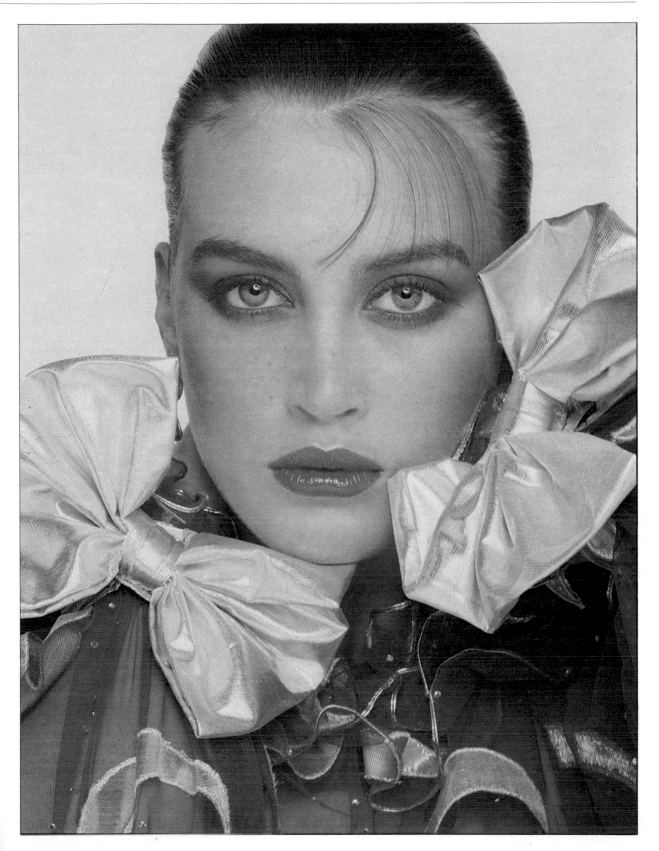

HAIR REMOVAL

Many people are concerned about unwanted facial and body hair, but it is, in fact, easy to deal with, and there are many ways of doing so. Most methods can be carried out at home and they are usually fairly inexpensive. Facial bleach, although not a hair-removing product, is useful for lightening facial or body hair if you do not actually want to get rid of it. There are several products on the market, made specifically to bleach facial and body hair, and they are available in most large chemists. Remember that bleaching hair will not remove it, it will just make it less obvious.

The speediest way of removing leg or under-arm hair is probably by shaving. However, the hair appears to grow through again very quickly and has blunt ends, which can feel very prickly, especially on the legs. If you do shave use a sharp blade and take a lot of care so that you do not cut yourself. *Never shave any hair on your face.*

Depilatory (hair-removing) creams are readily available in most big stores and chemists, and are a very good, if slightly messy, way of dealing with the removal of hair on your body and face. Although the re-growth of hair will seem nearly as rapid as after shaving, it tends to be a little less prickly since the hair is dissolved away (rather than cut) and therefore will reappear with its natural point.

If you only have to remove a few hairs from your face or body, you could try gently pulling them out with tweezers. Always pluck in the direction the hair is growing, so as not to break it off. It goes without saying that this should be done when the skin is clean. If you have hair in rather delicate areas and you do not want to remove it by another method, the best thing to do is just carefully snip it away with sharp nail scissors. This also goes for hair which grows out of moles. Under no circumstances should you pull out this hair, just snip it off.

One of the most efficient methods of hair removal is waxing. It can be done both on the face and body. Although it is usually reserved for the speedy removal of leg hair, it removes under-arm hair and bikini-line hair very well. If you are going on holiday and intend to spend a lot of time in a swim suit, it is a very good way of keeping your skin looking smoooth and hair-free while you are away. There are home waxing kits available but if you have the choice, you will probably find it quicker and less painful to have waxing done professionally.

Electrolysis

The only permanent way of removing any kind of unwanted hair is by electrolysis. There are several methods, but basically what happens is that a very fine needle is inserted into the hair follicle and a mild electric current is passed through it. This weakens the hair and it is lifted away with a pair of tweezers. Usually this process has to be repeated two or three times before the growth is deadened, but once this has been done, the hair will be gone forever. Electrolysis can only be done by a skilled operator and is, therefore, not particularly cheap. However, if superfluous hair is something that really worries you, then it is worth having electrolysis done. Do read all instruction leaflets very carefully and do not use strong creams or deodorants on your skin directly after any home treatment.

Unwanted hair worries many people but need not be a problem to remove given the home and clinical treatments now available.

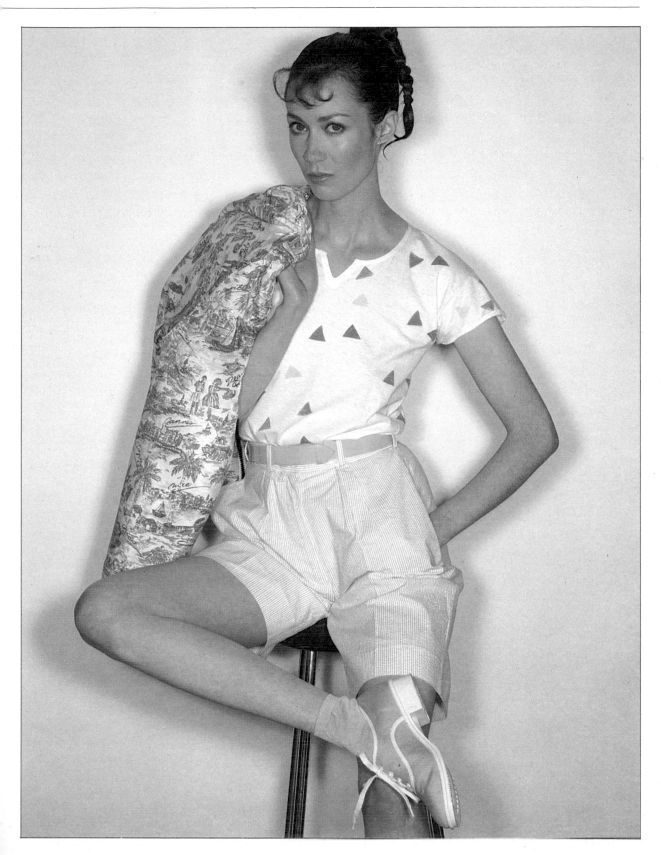

EYEBROWS

There is no such thing as the perfectly shaped eyebrow. Like every other facial feature, the best eyebrow for you is the one that most suits you. By all means be aware of changing trends in eyebrow shapes, or experiment with dyes for a deeper colour, but always remember that the right style for you probably lies somewhere between your natural line and the fashion of the moment.

Before you decide what is the best shape for you, pull your hair back off your face and take a long hard look at yourself. You may not have noticed your eyebrows for some time but they are one of the most mobile parts of your face, and usually provide a fairly accurate indication of your mood. It follows that, for instance, plucking them too much could make you look severe, or permanently surprised; letting them become overgrown could make you look scruffy or give your eyes a hooded, tired look.

Whatever you decide to do with your eyebrows, their own natural line should be taken into account. If it is a straight thin line, and the fashion is for thin arched brows, it is almost certainly a better idea to try gently to thin your eyebrows than to drastically alter their shape, which could look very odd and uneven. You can control the thickness of the line, and where it starts and ends, but remember that your eyebrow should not start any further back than the corner of your eye. With this in mind, decide what changes you want to make, and do not feel daunted. It is simple and straightforward once you have learned the technique. Mistakes, if you make them, will always grow out.

Plucking
When you come to pluck your eyebrows start with a clean face, without make-up. Tie your hair well back, make sure that you are by yourself and you are going to be undisturbed. Check that you are in a good light, whether it is natural or artificial, and you may find a magnifying mirror will be a great help. If you are short-sighted it will probably be essential. There are many tweezers on the market but you will probably find that tweezers which are not too big and have flat chisel-shaped ends are the easiest to use.

A good time to trim your eyebrows is either just after you have washed your face, and it is slightly warm and damp, or after a bath or shower. Alternatively you can use a piece of cotton wool or a face flannel wrung out in warm water to make the skin softer. Then wipe the skin with dilute surgical spirit to disinfect it, making sure that your tweezers are equally clean.

When plucking the hairs remember always to pull in the direction the hair is growing so that it does not break off. If you have not plucked your eyebrows before, just take out the hairs which may grow between your brows and then tidy up underneath the brow, remembering to follow the natural line.

When you have finished, clean the area again with dilute surgical spirit. If you then regularly tidy up your eyebrows and do not allow them to become straggly, you will never have to do the whole job again. Make sure when you have finished that your eyebrows match each other in thickness and length.

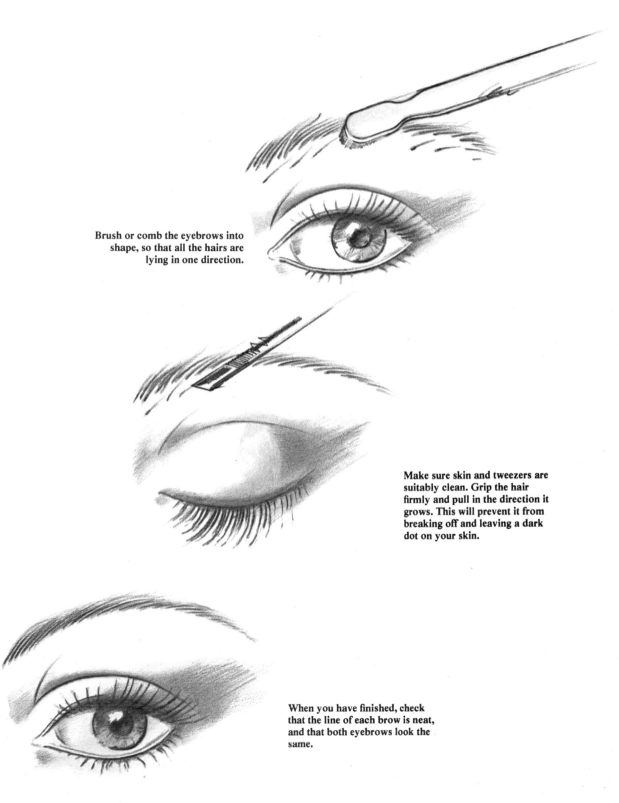

Brush or comb the eyebrows into shape, so that all the hairs are lying in one direction.

Make sure skin and tweezers are suitably clean. Grip the hair firmly and pull in the direction it grows. This will prevent it from breaking off and leaving a dark dot on your skin.

When you have finished, check that the line of each brow is neat, and that both eyebrows look the same.

HOLIDAY SKIN

Everyone would like to look good on holiday and there is usually a little extra time before going away to collect the things you need and to prepare yourself. Sometimes the thought of exposing your very white skin to the sun is a rather daunting prospect, particularly if it has suffered from the effects of a hard winter. The sun seems to emphasize a dull complexion and hitherto unnoticed blemishes and blackheads may appear. A thorough cleansing to remove deep-seated grime is a great facial refresher. You can do this at home by cleansing thoroughly, and then gently steaming your face over a bowl of warm water into which you have thrown a handful of sweet smelling herbs and flowers such as camomile or lavender. Then cleanse again, and apply a face mask which is suitable for your skin type.

If you have blackheads, you can try removing them after steaming, when the skin is very soft and supple. First, disinfect your skin and fingers by lightly wiping them and the problem area with diluted surgical spirit and cover the tips of your fingers with tissue. Then gently squeeze the blackheads. *Never* try to force out a stubborn blemish – you will only damage the surrounding tissue and leave a big red mark on your skin. After this treatment you should apply a face mask.

A very efficient way of getting your skin really clean is to have a professional facial. This is also very relaxing and will put you in a holiday mood. If you are very fair, you could use your time at the beauticians to have your eyelashes dyed. This can be done at home using one of the proprietary brands (read the instructions carefully), but having someone else do it for you means that they can put the dye

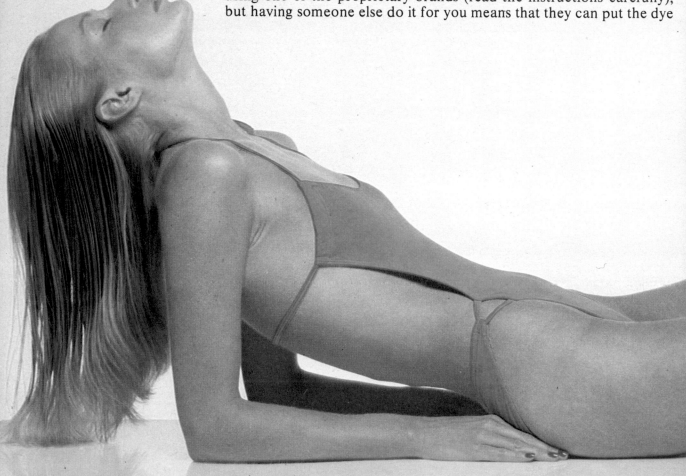

right to the roots of the lashes. If you prefer fuzz-free legs and you are not using a hair-removing cream or waxing them yourself, remember to make an appointment for them to be waxed a couple of days before you go away.

You may notice that your feet, which have been covered up all winter long do not look very good in sandals. There are various ways of smoothing off hard skin, a pumice stone probably being the cheapest and most effective home treatment, but for good-looking, comfortable feet, treat yourself to a visit to the chiropodist, followed by a pedicure.

Your hands, although not calloused like your feet, will probably benefit from a little extra attention. Have a professional manicure or give yourself a manicure at home. If your hands feel very dry, and the nails and cuticles do not seem in very good condition, try soaking the finger tips in warm olive oil for a few minutes, and then rub the residue of the oil, along with some rich hand cream, into the hands. Leave this on as long as possible and repeat as often as you can.

There are lots of products available which make the skin appear lightly tanned. They are very useful for really pale-skinned people who have to take the first days of a sun and sea holiday very carefully, and hate the thought of being the whitest thing on the beach! Read the instructions about how to apply very thoroughly, for if not used properly you can end up with streaky skin and orange knees and elbows. Fake tan lasts two or three days, but you can keep re-applying it as long as you need to or until you become lightly tanned. Fake tans *do not*

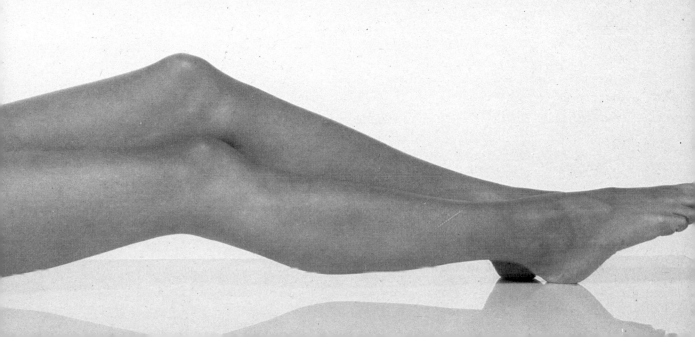

protect you from burning in the sun. All they do is make the skin slightly brown. It is essential that you use a sun screen to filter out the harmful rays as well. You can prepare your skin for long periods of sun-bathing by having a course of treatments in a solarium or on a sun bed. These are also very useful for helping your tan to last slightly longer after your holidays.

If you are having a beach holiday, it is likely that you will be exposing a great deal of your body to the sun, and most of it will not have been exposed to the elements for the previous nine or ten months. Therefore, it is important that you are very careful for the first two or three days and that you use enough sun cream. Frequent applications of the correct sun product for your skin type does not stop you from tanning, in fact it encourages it, but it does stop you from burning.

Under nearly all circumstances it is not a good idea to sun your face. This soon encourages lines and wrinkles and you will find that there is usually enough reflected sunlight around to give your face colour. If you want your face to be darker it is better to boost up the colour artificially with a fake tan. Be very wary of over-exposing your shoulders, backs of legs, nose, soles of feet or eyelids. Remember that if you spend a lot of time in the sea you may still get burned because the sun's rays will penetrate the water. If you are snorkelling, it is a good idea to wear a T-shirt.

To really protect your face or any sensitive areas of the body there are special sun-block creams on the market which stop all the ultra-

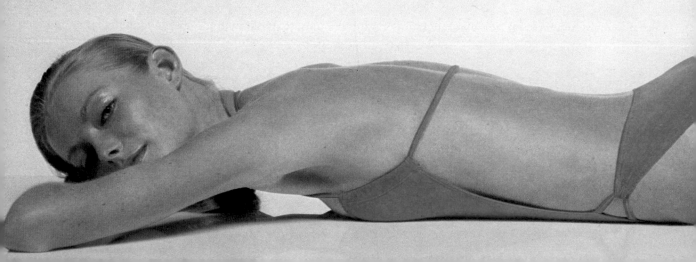

violet light from reaching your skin. These are particularly useful for people who have very fair skins. The main rule to remember is have a healthy respect for the sun, especially at midday, and do not spoil your holiday by getting burned.

If you are a winter-sports fan, a big danger area for you is your face. Always use a good sun screen, and apply moisturiser lavishly when you have finished skiing. Cover your face as much as you can when out in the snow, and try to protect the more sensitive areas of eyes and lips by using eye goggles or sunglasses and one of the lip protection products. If you are skiing in fairly warm weather and are wearing light clothing such as T-shirts, do not forget that although the wind may make you feel quite cool whilst skiing down the slopes, you can still get badly burned. The same applies to those who intend to spend time aboard a boat. Sea breezes are very misleading and if you do not take the proper precautions you can feel very sore and uncomfortable when going indoors after a day on the water.

A small portion of nearly everyone's holidays is spent sight-seeing and though you may be dressed and spending most of the day walking around, you should still make sure that the tops of your shoulders, face, arms and legs are properly protected by the use of sun cream.

If you do manage to burn yourself in the sun there are many after-sun lotions available. They cool down the surface of the skin and help to replace some of the lost moisture. You should certainly use a body lotion at the end of each day to keep your skin smooth and supple.

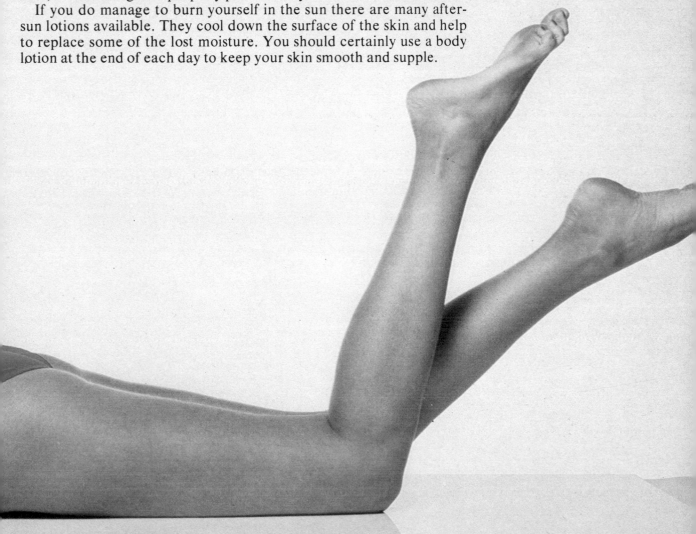

Holiday make-up

The following are a few tips for holiday make-up. Rather than toasting it in the sun, use a light tanning gel or liquid on your face, not heavy foundation. Use only the very thinnest of foundations if you need one, or perhaps just a concealer stick on any discoloured areas. Before moisturising, to cool your skin, you can give it a light spray of mineral water. This is very refreshing. Try using non-crease eye-shadows in hot weather, and lipsticks which are not too thin since they seem to disappear very quickly in the heat.

However much you like the sun, do not put too much emphasis on tanning during your holiday and risk burning your skin. With a sensible tanning programme even the fairest skin is likely to be tanned after a two-week holiday. You do not have to lie out in the sun for eight hours every day and run the risk of burning yourself. Nothing is worse than having to stay indoors because you have overdone it.

Sun screens

Creams, oils and lotions that protect the skin from burning in the sun, are to be found in many forms. Sun-screen products *do not* prevent your skin from becoming tanned, what they do is screen out the harmful rays of the sun and stop you from burning. Everyone, unless they spend most of their time in the sun and have a natural build-up of melanin (the pigment in your skin which makes it go brown) must use some form of sun screen. Even people with dark oily skins need protection of some kind. Ordinary oils, such as olive oil or baby oil, *do not* protect you. On the contrary, using an oil in the sun you more or less 'fry' your skin. Oils are quite good, however, used as lubricants after sunbathing.

Sun oils are best left to those people with darker skins. Clear, tinted liquids are good for people who have very greasy or spotty skins. Sun milks and lotions, which are also sometimes slightly tinted to give the impression of a very light tan, are suitable for normal-to-dry skins, as are the thicker richer creams. For children, and people with fair or sensitive skins there are special screening creams which block out the sun's harmful rays completely. These products are very good for putting on any extremely sensitive areas which are prone to burning, such as the nose.

Many sun products are numbered. The numbering system is not uniform but it generally means that the higher the number the more protection it affords. For prolonged periods of sunbathing use the higher numbers first until your natural tan has started to build up. For example, if you are a light-skinned person, you should use a cream or lotion with a SPF (sun protection factor) of say 6 or 8 for the first two or three days, then as your skin begins to tan you should use a filter factor 3 or 4 and perhaps in the last four or five days when you already have a good tan a filter factor of 2 or 3 would be sufficient. If you are anything other than naturally dark-skinned do not use the oil products. Because the numbering is not consistent across the many brands of sun screens, please read the labels very carefully. Never forget that children will invariably need a higher SPF factor for a longer period than the average adult. Apply sun-screen products frequently.

If you tan sensibly while on holiday and do not get burnt, your tan will last you longer when you come home.

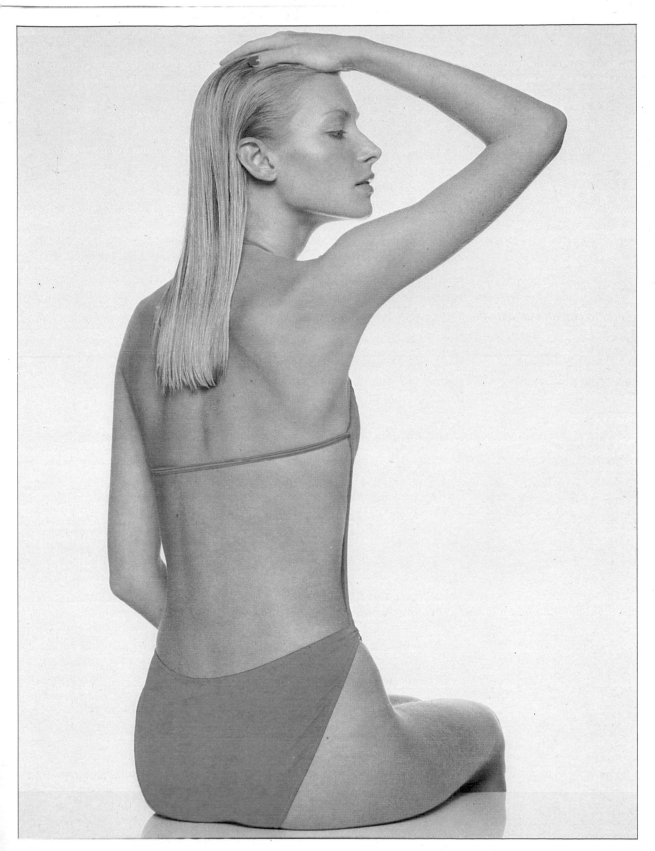

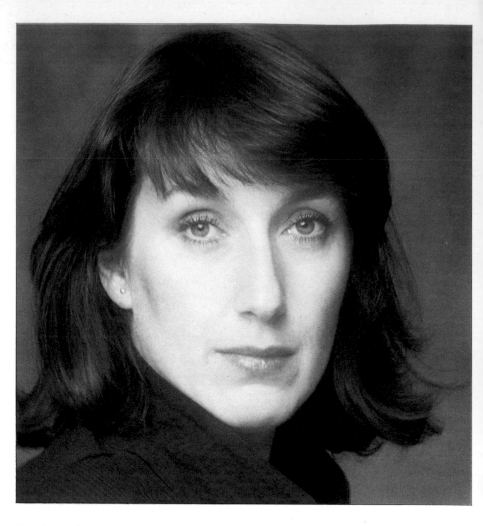

Barbara Daly is responsible for much new thought in face-making in Britain. Her work is regularly seen in *Vogue, Harpers and Queen* and other fashion magazines. She creates faces for feature films, such as *A Clockwork Orange* and *Barry Lyndon*, and for television commercials. Barbara has built up an international reputation for the artistry and imagination she has brought to her work as a make-up designer.

ACKNOWLEDGEMENTS

There is no word strong enough for me to express how grateful I am to everyone who contributed to the programme and this book and helped in so many ways. A special thank-you to Sam and to Tony Essam, John Swannell, Alexander Vethers, John Frieda, Annabel Hodin, Neil Tennant, Nina Burr, Tim Moores and everyone at Thames, not forgetting Sue Davies who never forgot anything – thank you.

Love

Barbara